A Colour Atlas of
Liver
Disease

Dame Sheila Sherlock

DBE, MD, DSc(NY)(Hon), FRCP, FRCP(E), FRCCP(Hon),
FRCP(I)(Hon), FACP(Hon)

Professor of Medicine and Chairman of
Department of Medicine in the
University of London at the
Royal Free Hospital School of Medicine

John A. Summerfield

MD, MRCP

Lecturer in Medicine at the
Royal Free Hospital School of Medicine

Wolfe Medical Publications Ltd

Acknowledgements

We are deeply indebted to Dr R. Dick (Consultant Radiologist) and Professor P. J. Scheuer (Professor of Histopathology), at the Royal Free Hospital, for their help and advice. In addition, Dr R. Dick provided many of the radiological illustrations and Professor P. J. Scheuer much of the histological material. We are very grateful for the many pictures provided by Mr J. Agnew and Mr J. Wood (Senior Physicists), Dr L. Berger (Consultant Radiologist) and Professor K. E. F. Hobbs (Professor of Surgery).

We also thank our past and present colleagues at the Royal Postgraduate Medical School and the Royal Free Hospital, including Dr Bengt Arborgh, Dr G. Chadwick, Dr J. Dooley, Dr E. Elias, Miss Phyllis George, Dr Angela Gorman, Dr R. Hunt, Dr D. Jewell, Dr A. P. Kirk, Dr T. Lyssiotis, Dr N. McIntyre, Mr S. Parbhoo and Dr G. Smith-Laing.

This Atlas could not have been compiled without the generous help of many other friends and colleagues, including Dr June Almeida, Wellcome Research Laboratories, Kent, Dr S. Bender, Dr K. Hübner and Dr P. Rottger, Frankfurt, F.R.G., Professor M. J. Clarkson, Liverpool School of Tropical Medicine, Liverpool, Major-General J. C. Crook, Ministry of Defence, London, Professor G. M. Edington and Dr Y. M. Fakunle, Zaria, Nigeria, Dr S. V. Feinman, Toronto, Canada, Dr J. Galambos and Dr Hersh, Atlanta, U.S.A., Mr B. Hawkes, Sittingbourne, Kent, Professor M. S. R. Hutt, St Thomas's Hospital, London, Professor Prayat Laksanaphuk, Bangkok, Thailand, Dr F. Margolin and Dr J. Bennington, San Francisco, U.S.A., Professor G. A. Martini, Marburg, F.R.G., Professor W. Peters, Liverpool School of Tropical Medicine, Liverpool, Dr W. Pipatnagul, Bangkok, Thailand, Dr M. F. Sorrell, Omaha, U.S.A., Dr G. Whelan, Melbourne, Australia, Dr E. Williams, Pembrokeshire, Wales and Professor A. W. Woodruff, London School of Tropical Medicine and Hygiene, London.

Finally, we thank Mr Cedric C. Gilson (Director) and his colleagues, Mrs Ruth M. Eastwood, Mr Michael J. Graham, Miss Julie M. Phipps, Mr Jozef Pollak and Mrs Ann K. Sym of the Department of Medical Illustration at the Royal Free Hospital for the excellent photographic work, Miss Janice Cox for the artwork and Mrs Jean Fulcher for typing the manuscript.

Contents

Preface

Recent advances in hepatology have made it even more essential to be familiar with the clinical signs and pathology of liver disease. The correct management of patients is becoming increasingly dependent on a precise diagnosis. Our aim in this Atlas has been to compile an up-to-date and comprehensive collection of the physical signs, pathology and investigations of liver disease. This format has permitted the collection of a much larger number of high quality colour photographs than is normally possible in standard textbooks. However the Atlas should be used as a companion to the standard textbooks on the subject. For this reason the legends to the pictures have been ruthlessly pruned to keep them short; the pictures should speak for themselves. The book begins with a general chapter on the examination of the liver and the signs of liver disease. Subsequent chapters deal with the major groups of diseases affecting the liver, with their special signs.

We hope that clinical medical students and candidates for higher examinations, both medical and surgical, will find the Atlas a useful adjunct to their studies. General physicians, surgeons and gastro-enterologists will find a comprehensive survey of the signs of hepatology, including rare conditions that they will only occasionally encounter.

For systematic accounts, in particular of disease mechanisms and treatment, readers are recommended to consult the standard texts on liver disease, including Sherlock, S., *Diseases of the Liver and Biliary System,* Fifth Edition 1975, Blackwell Scientific Publications and Lippincott; Schiff, L., *Diseases of the Liver,* Fourth Edition 1975, Lippincott; Scheuer, P. J., *Liver Biopsy Interpretation,* Third Edition to be published in 1980, Baillière Tindall.

It is hoped that this book will withstand the barriers of language and time. The message should be understood by those whose first language is not English and after many current theories of disease and methods of investigation and treatment have been long forgotten.

NORMAL VALUES

Serum total bilirubin 0.3–1.0mg/100ml
                                5–17μmol/l
Serum aspartate transaminase (SGOT) 5–15iU/l
Prothrombin time 11–14 seconds

All the scales shown are in centimetres.

The magnification factors of histological slides
refer to the original 35mm colour transparencies.

1. Clinical examination of the liver and biliary system

Examination of the liver

1. The normal liver, the largest organ in the body, weighs about 1.5kg. The upper border is at the level of the 5th rib, the lower border lies under the costal margin on the right. The lower edge is usually palpable in deep inspiration when the liver moves downwards. The upper border is defined by heavy percussion. Light percussion together with palpation will identify the lower border. An estimate of liver size can be obtained from the vertical length of dullness to percussion in the right mid clavicular line (usually 12–15cm). It is reduced in cirrhosis and fulminant hepatitis and is important in monitoring progress. Routine examination of the liver must include auscultation for friction rubs. These may be due to a recent liver biopsy or to a tumour. Arterial bruits may be related to acute alcoholic hepatitis or to primary liver cell cancer. Venous hums can be due to portal hypertension. The spleen is rarely palpable in health.

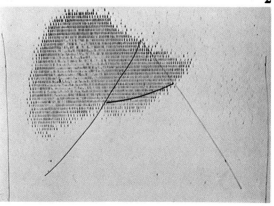

2. Isotope scan of the liver. An intravenous injection of the gamma emitting isotope [99]technetium is taken up by the reticulo-endothelial cells of the liver. The normal scan shows a uniform distribution of the isotope throughout the liver; no isotope uptake is seen in the spleen. Filling defects larger than about 2cm will be shown. In special circumstances other isotopes are employed. [67]Gallium citrate is taken up by primary liver cell cancers and granulocytes in the walls of abscesses. These lesions give filling defects with a [99]technetium scan.

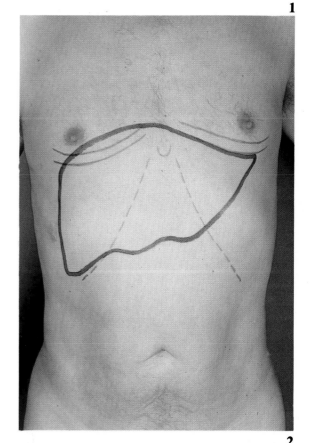

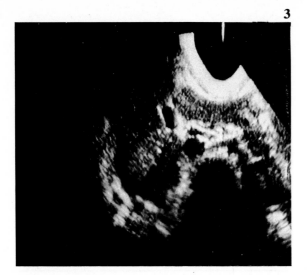

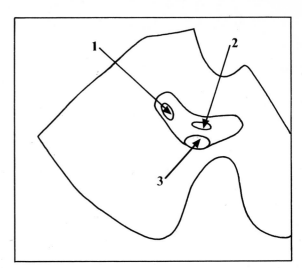

3. Grey scale ultrasonography reveals the liver as a large trans-sonic area. In addition, the portal vein (1), inferior vena cava (2) and aorta (3) are shown. The normal biliary system is not seen. This non-invasive technique also permits study of the portal venous system and the pancreas.

4. Computerised tomography of the liver shows the liver (1) and spleen (2) clearly. The line drawing at the top shows the level at which this CAT scan was taken. The scan also shows a vertebral body (3), aorta (4), pancreas (5) and stomach (6).

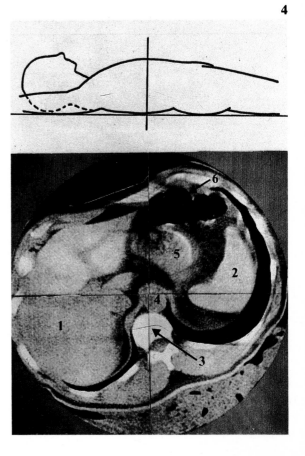

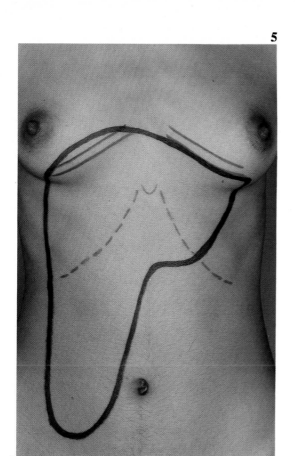

5

5. Riedel's lobe. The right lobe of the liver is enlarged by a tongue-like extension. This anatomical variation is more common in women and is of no consequence. It may be mistaken for a liver tumour or an enlarged right kidney.

6

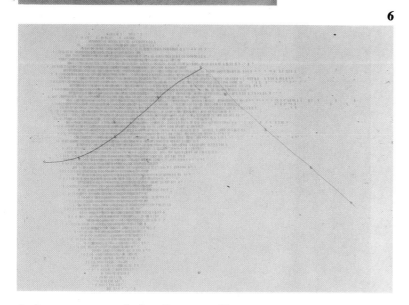

6. Isotope scan of the liver readily reveals a Riedel's lobe in this patient.

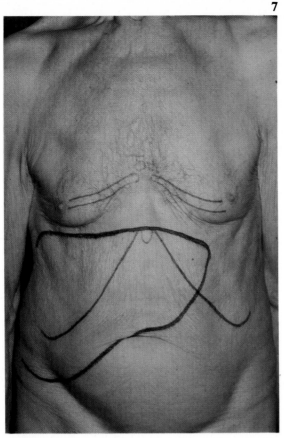

7. The liver in emphysema. Diseases, such as emphysema, which increase the volume of the chest may displace the liver downwards so that its lower edge is easily palpable. Percussion of the upper border of the liver will reveal that the liver is not enlarged. Late in the course of emphysema hepatomegaly is common, due to right heart failure.

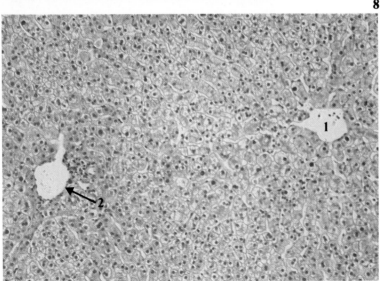

8. Liver biopsy. The normal liver consists of sheets of hepatocytes, supported by a reticulin framework, separating hepatic veins in the centre from portal tracts at the periphery of the lobule. The *Haematoxylin and Eosin* stain (×*40*) shows the relationship between the hepatic veins (1) and portal tracts (2).

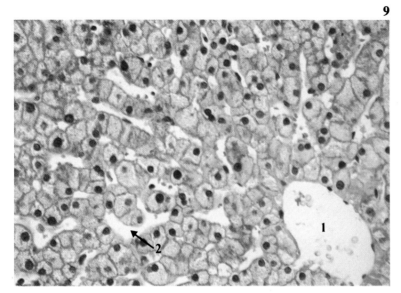

9. Hepatic veins (1) drain the sinusoids (2) which perfuse the sheets of hepatocytes. *(H. & E. ×140)*

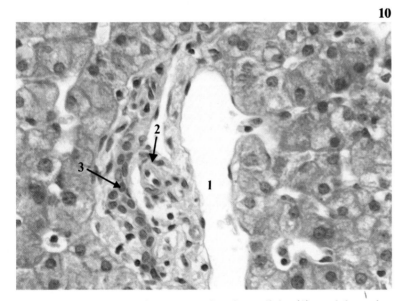

10. Portal tract contains a portal vein radicle (1) and hepatic arteriole (2) which supply the hepatic sinusoids and a small bile duct (3) draining the biliary canaliculi which traverse the surface of each hepatocyte. *(H. & E. ×160)*

Jaundice

11. Mild jaundice (serum bilirubin 3mg/100ml; 51 μmol/l). Jaundice is due to staining of the tissues with bilirubin and possibly other pigments such as biliverdin. It is first detected in the sclera of the eye where it is strongly bound by the abundant elastic tissue. Accumulation of bilirubin may result from either overproduction (haemolytic anaemias) or reduced excretion (liver cell or biliary disease). This patient had a cancer of the common hepatic duct.

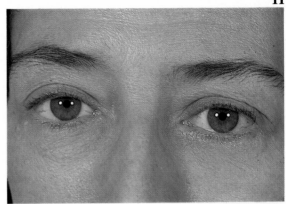

12. Severe jaundice (serum bilirubin 16mg/100ml; 272 μmol/l). As jaundice deepens the skin becomes progressively more pigmented, although paralysed and oedematous areas are usually spared. In severe jaundice all tissues except the brain become pigmented and bilirubin appears in the urine, sweat, semen and tears. Rarely in severe jaundice bilirubin in the eye results in yellow vision (xanthopsia). In the newborn unconjugated bilirubin may enter the central nervous system and accumulate in the basal ganglia (kernicterus). Jaundice may be classified into three main groups: haemolytic, hepatocellular (hepatitic) and cholestatic (biliary obstruction). This patient had primary biliary cirrhosis where the jaundice is of predominantly cholestatic (biliary obstructive) type. The colour of the jaundice differs in the three types.

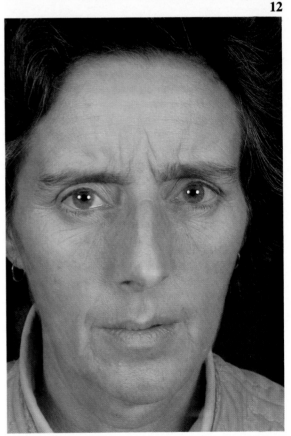

13. Haemolytic jaundice (serum bilirubin 4mg/100ml; 68 μmol/l) in a young woman with autoimmune haemolytic anaemia. Haemolytic jaundice has a light lemon yellow colour and is due to overproduction of bilirubin. The serum total bilirubin level rarely exceeds 5mg/100ml (85 μmol/l) and the circulating bilirubin is mainly unconjugated (non-esterified).

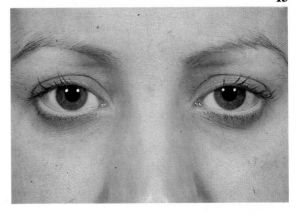

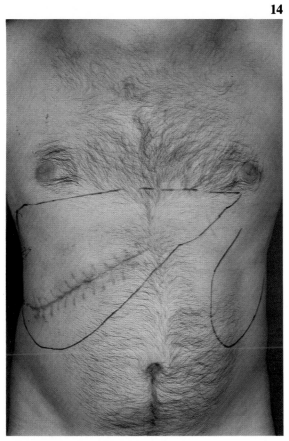

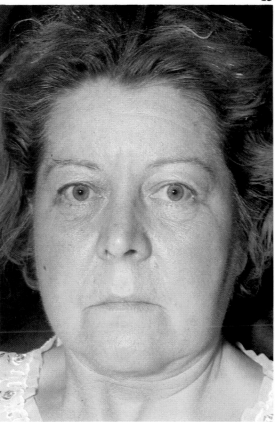

14. Hepato-splenomegaly usually accompanies haemolytic jaundice. This man, with chronic auto-immune haemolytic anaemia, had previously had his gall bladder removed because it contained pigment gallstones.

15. Hepatitic jaundice is usually of orange yellow colour as shown in this patient with a drug-induced hepatitis due to isoniazid; the total serum bilirubin was 18mg/100ml (306μmol/l). The liver was not enlarged.

16. Alcoholic hepatitis. The orange yellow colour of hepatitic jaundice is also evident in this patient with alcoholic hepatitis. The serum total bilirubin concentration was 22mg/100ml (374µmol/l). The liver was enlarged due to infiltration with fat. In addition histology showed liver cell necrosis and cellular infiltration, typical of alcoholic hepatitis.

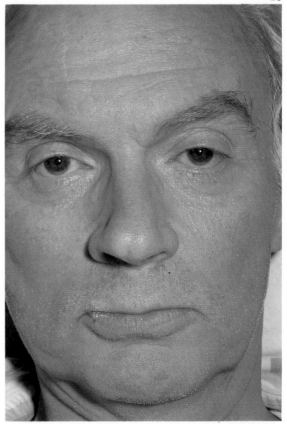

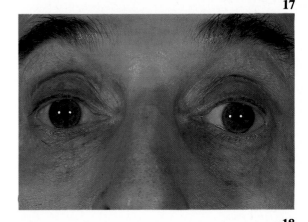

17. Cholestatic jaundice has a greenish yellow colour. The patient had a carcinoma of the head of the pancreas which resulted in obstruction of the common bile duct. The serum total bilirubin level was 15mg/100ml (255µmol/l).

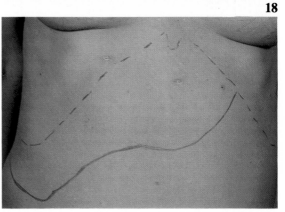

18. Hepatomegaly is an important sign of cholestasis due to obstructed bile ducts. Scratch marks were seen on the abdominal wall due to pruritus (itching).

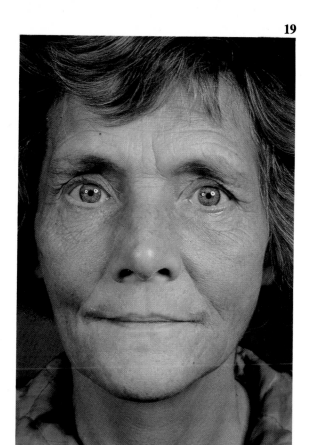

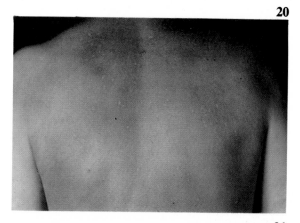

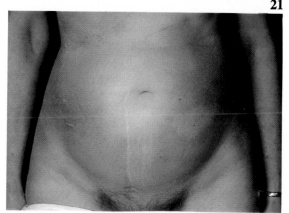

19–21. Pigmentation of the skin follows prolonged cholestatic jaundice. The grey or brown pigmentation is due to melanin in the skin. This European patient had long standing cholestasis due to primary biliary cirrhosis. Careful camouflage make-up is necessary to hide the progressive pigmentation.

On the back (**20**) an area in a butterfly distribution may escape pigmentation. This butterfly sign is attributed to the patient being unable to scratch that area. Pigmentation of the skin in chronic cholestasis is found all over the body. This patient's abdomen is heavily pigmented but old scars are spared.

22. Urine in jaundice. In jaundiced patients the normal urine (1) is darkened by the renal excretion of bile pigments. In cholestasis conjugated bilirubin in urine confers a greeny yellow colour (2). In haemolysis and cirrhosis (3) the urine is a warm orange colour due to urobilin. The excretion of bile pigment falls with recovery or the onset of renal failure.

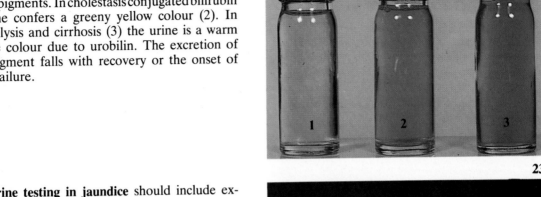

23. Urine testing in jaundice should include examination for conjugated bilirubin (by Ictotest) and urobilinogen (by Urobilistix or Ehrlich's aldehyde reagent). Normal urine (1) contains neither pigment. Cholestatic urine (2) contains conjugated bilirubin, shown by the purple ring around the Ictotest tablet, but no urobilinogen because bilirubin is not present in the gut contents. In haemolysis or cirrhosis (3) there is no bilirubin, but an excess amount of urobilinogen indicated by the brown colour of the Urobilistix, because bilirubin is excreted into the gut and is converted to urobilinogen which is reabsorbed. In haemolysis the excess urobilinogenuria is due to increased production in the gut. In cirrhosis it is caused by failure of the liver to excrete the normal load of reabsorbed urobilinogen.

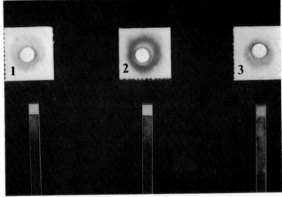

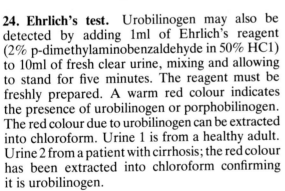

24. Ehrlich's test. Urobilinogen may also be detected by adding 1ml of Ehrlich's reagent (2% p-dimethylaminobenzaldehyde in 50% HC1) to 10ml of fresh clear urine, mixing and allowing to stand for five minutes. The reagent must be freshly prepared. A warm red colour indicates the presence of urobilinogen or porphobilinogen. The red colour due to urobilinogen can be extracted into chloroform. Urine 1 is from a healthy adult. Urine 2 from a patient with cirrhosis; the red colour has been extracted into chloroform confirming it is urobilinogen.

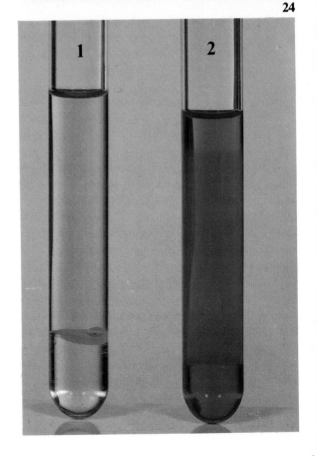

25. The stools in jaundice are pale because there is obstruction to the biliary excretion of bilirubin pigments. The degree of pallor depends on the severity of biliary obstruction, being most marked in cholestatic jaundice. These are the faeces of a patient with complete bile duct obstruction due to a bile duct carcinoma. Cancers of the ampulla of Vater give a 'silver' stool due to the presence of blood in addition to lack of bile pigments. In haemolysis the stools are darker than normal due to increased red cell destruction and bilirubin formation.

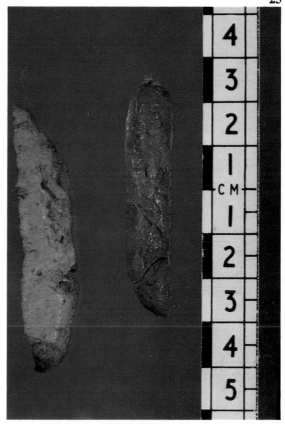

26. Mepacrine treatment for malaria or tapeworms can result in yellow discoloration of the skin which may mimic that due to jaundice. However, unlike jaundice, the ocular sclera are not pigmented. Carotenaemia can cause an orange-yellow skin discoloration that may be confused with jaundice.

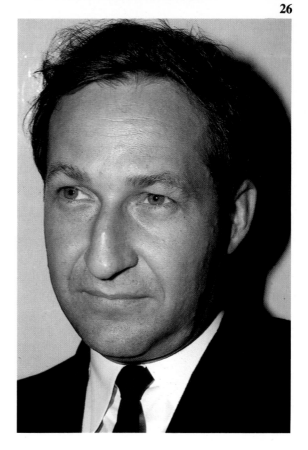

Signs in liver disease

27. Spider naevi (vascular spiders) are vascular skin lesions. These are supplied by a central arteriole and they blanch if it is occluded with a pinhead. Palpation of larger spiders may reveal pulsation due to the arteriolar dilatation.

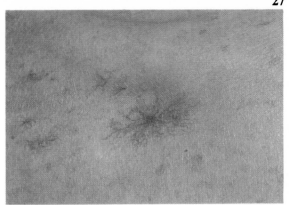

28. Spider naevi are characteristically surrounded by a pale area or white spot (see also **32**). The pale areas are clearly seen on the hand of this young girl with chronic active hepatitis. Spider naevi occur in the distribution of the superior vena cava, the chest above the nipples, face, arms and hands.

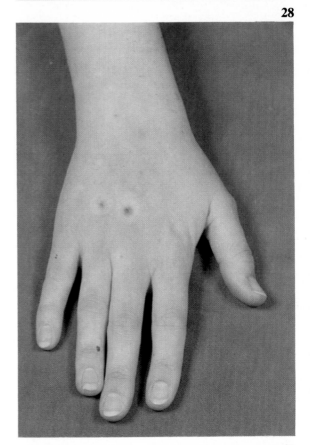

29. Spider naevi. One or two spider naevi may be found in health, especially during pregnancy or in childhood. The later appearance of such lesions and their increase in size indicates chronic liver disease, as on the neck of this patient with alcoholic cirrhosis.

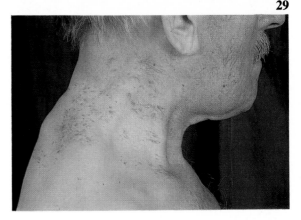

30. Campbell de Morgan spots must be distinguished from spider naevi. These bright red discrete punctate spots are 1–2mm in diameter. Campbell de Morgan spots are found mainly on the chest and abdomen, especially as age advances. They are of no significance.

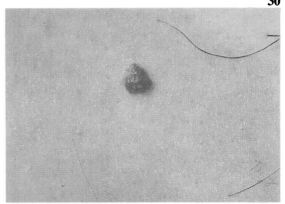

31. Paper money skin describes the random distribution of fine threadlike blood vessels just under the skin, seen here on the face of a patient with alcoholic hepatitis. Paper money skin occurs in the same distribution as spider naevi and indicates chronic liver disease. It is named after the silk threads in American dollar bills.

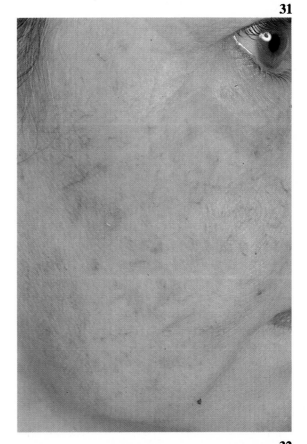

32. White spots develop on the arms, buttocks and legs in patients with chronic liver disease, especially when the skin is cold. In the centre of each white spot is an arteriole which later develops into a spider naevus. This patient had chronic active hepatitis. They are also seen in pregnancy.

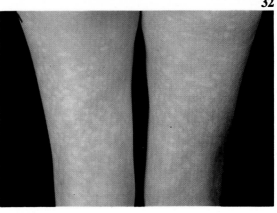

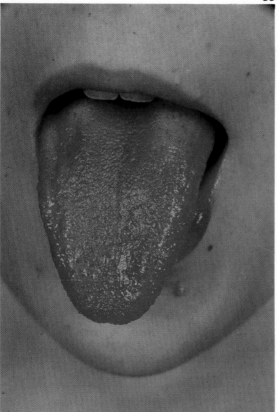

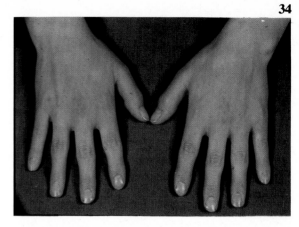

33, 34. Central cyanosis is due to vasodilatation
and arteriovenous shunting in the lungs. It may be
demonstrated in decompensated cirrhosis. An
extreme example is shown in this young woman
in the late stages of chronic active hepatitis. Her
hands (**34**) are also cyanosed. The chronic cyanosis
has resulted in clubbing of her fingers.

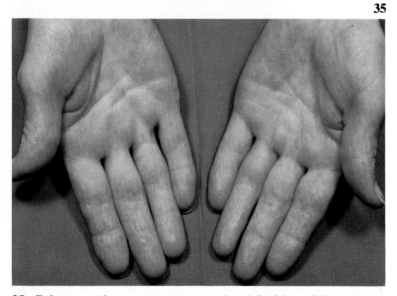

35. Palmar erythema, an exaggerated red flushing of the palms,
affects especially the thenar and hypothenar eminences and the
bases of the fingers. It fades on pressure. Although a useful sign
of chronic liver disease, it is also seen in pregnancy, thyrotoxicosis,
bronchial carcinoma and as a genetically determined abnormality.

36. **Red soles** of the feet may also be seen when there is palmar erythema of the hands. This patient suffered from alcoholic cirrhosis.

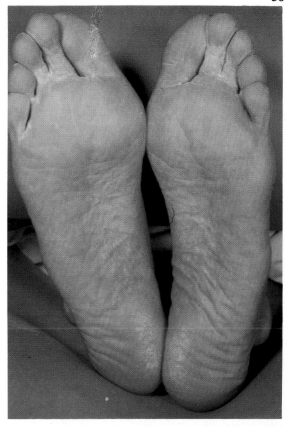

37. **White nails** are present in most patients with cirrhosis. The tip of the nail remains pink and in severe cases, such as this patient with primary biliary cirrhosis, the lunula of the nail disappears. Clubbing of the fingers in this patient is also seen in chronic cholestasis.

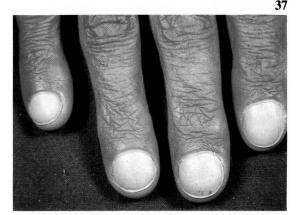

38. Gynaecomastia or enlargement of the breasts is sometimes seen in males with cirrhosis. The diagnosis can only be made if there is palpable enlargement of breast tissue. The breasts may be tender and the areolar pigmented. There is usually associated diminished libido and testicular atrophy. Gynaecomastia is common in alcoholic cirrhosis but is also found in men with chronic active hepatitis. Note the absent body hair, jaundice and spider naevi in this young man with chronic active hepatitis. Spironolactone therapy is a very frequent cause of gynaecomastia in male patients with cirrhosis and ascites. In women with chronic liver disease breast atrophy and amenorrhoea occur.

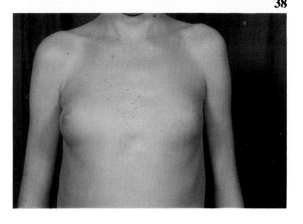

39. Weight loss is a feature of advanced chronic liver disease. Severe weight loss with an enlarged, hard, irregular liver suggests a malignant tumour in the liver as illustrated by this patient who suffered from primary liver cell cancer. More common causes of secondary deposits in the liver are metastases from cancer of the breast, bronchus, stomach, pancreas, colon or thyroid. In the patient illustrated note the cachectic facies and profound loss of muscle bulk.

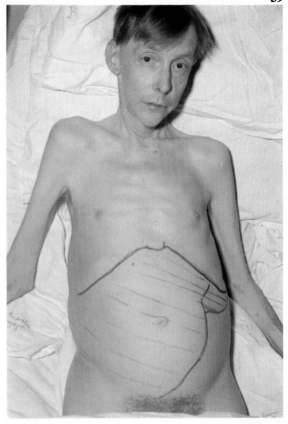

40. Spontaneous bruising around the eye of this cirrhotic patient is caused by a clotting defect due to the failure of hepatic synthesis of clotting factors.

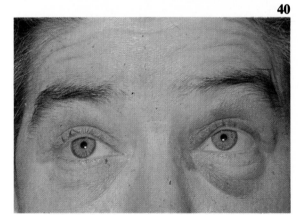

41. Venepuncture sites. Excessive bruising around venepuncture sites is another important sign of a clotting disorder in liver disease. This patient had fulminant hepatitis and a prothrombin time prolonged more than 10 seconds over control values after intramuscular vitamin K therapy.

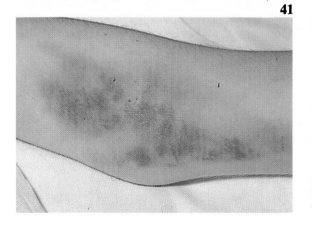

42. Arterial puncture in this patient with fulminant hepatic failure has resulted in massive extravasation of blood, despite prolonged pressure over the puncture site. This is due to the profound clotting disorder following failure to synthesise clotting factors.

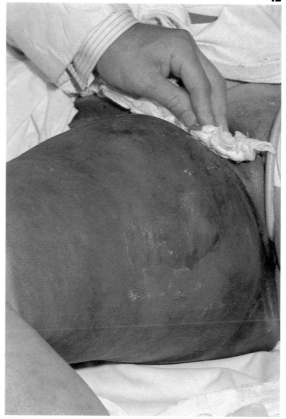

43. Spontaneous ecchymoses become widespread late in the course of hepatic failure and this is a poor prognostic sign. This man with fulminant viral hepatitis died three hours later.

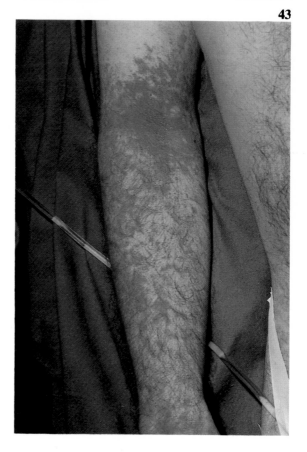

44. Hepatic coma is a late stage of acute hepatic failure and of chronic liver disease. Personality changes, sleepiness and a day-night reversal of sleep patterns are early features. Mania and violent screaming attacks are common in children. Other signs include fetor, a coarse, flapping tremor and increased tendon reflexes with upgoing plantar responses. Hepatic coma is easily confused with encephalitis and other metabolic causes. This young girl is in hepatic coma due to fulminant type B viral hepatitis. Stimulation of her achilles tendon has resulted in the posture of decerebrate rigidity. The arms are internally rotated at the shoulders and extended at the elbows. The legs are extended and adducted. This is usually a poor prognostic sign appearing late in the course of acute hepatic coma.

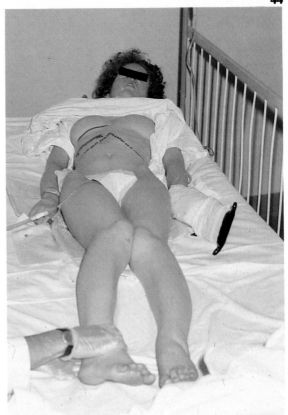

45. 'Doll's eye' movement, another grave sign of brain stem dysfunction, is present in the patient shown in **44**. The eyes remain fixed as the head is moved. However these signs, severe as they are, are not always incompatible with survival. This patient recovered completely after careful supportive management.

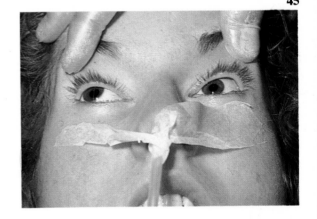

46. Pruritus occurs in cholestatic liver disease. Although usually generalised, the palms and soles are most affected. The symptom may become intolerable in chronic cholestasis, such as this patient with primary biliary cirrhosis, resulting in severe excoriations.

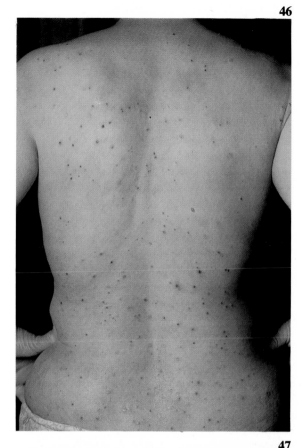

47. Xanthomas develop in prolonged cholestasis. These consist histologically of foamy cells full of cholesterol. They are associated with an elevated serum cholesterol concentration. Xanthomas first develop around the eye (xanthelasma), starting at the inner canthus and spreading laterally. Later xanthomas appear on extensor surfaces, particularly elbows, buttocks, palms, neck, chest and back.

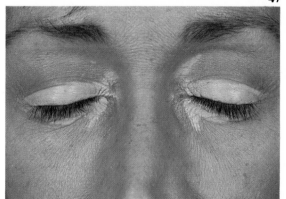

48. Finger clubbing is a feature of chronic cholestasis. This patient has primary biliary cirrhosis.

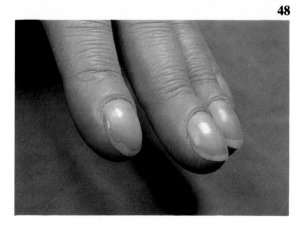

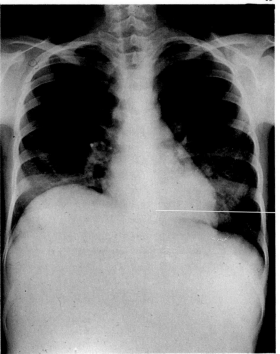

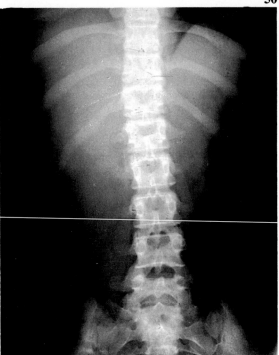

49. Chest x-ray is an essential part of the investigation of a patient with liver disease. An enlarged liver elevates the right hemidiaphragm in this patient with primary liver cell cancer. A metastasis is present in the right lower zone of the lung.

50. Abdominal x-ray from the same patient shows a grossly enlarged liver filling the right side of the abdomen. The ribs on the right have been spread apart by the enlarged liver. The spleen is not visible. An abdominal x-ray is useful for estimating liver and spleen size and may provide other information, including calcification in the liver, pancreas or gallstones, air in the biliary tree and ascites.

Ascites

51. Ascites represents the accumulation of fluid in the abdomen. When due to liver disease the cause is either local, such as a tumour, or liver cell failure with portal hypertension. This patient with decompensated alcoholic cirrhosis has moderate ascites. The abdomen is distended, especially in the flanks. The distance between the umbilicus and the symphysis pubis appears diminished and the umbilicus is everted.

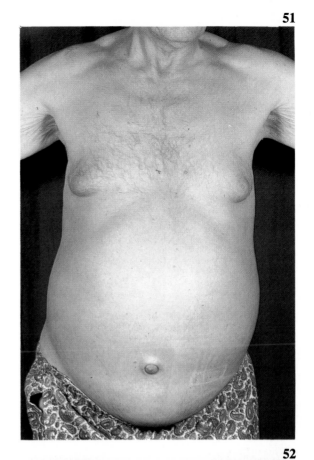

52. Ascites. The lateral view of this patient shows the maximum circumference of the abdomen is above the umbilicus which is everted. Dullness to percussion is maximal in the flanks but shifts on movement. There is marked muscle wasting and gynaecomastia.

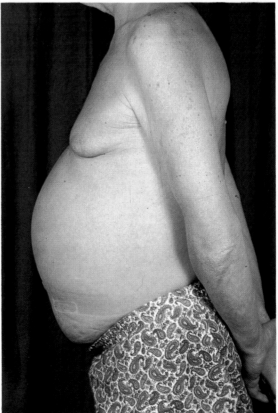

53. Gross ascites in a Persian man with cirrhosis due to chronic viral hepatitis (type B). The umbilicus has herniated and the scrotum is distended with fluid. The veins on his upper abdomen and chest represent portal-systemic venous collaterals and signify portal hypertension.

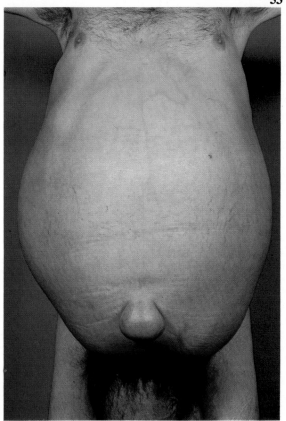

54. Ascites in a child with cirrhosis. The profound muscle wasting is apparent in the limbs and buttocks. Growth in this four-year-old child is retarded.

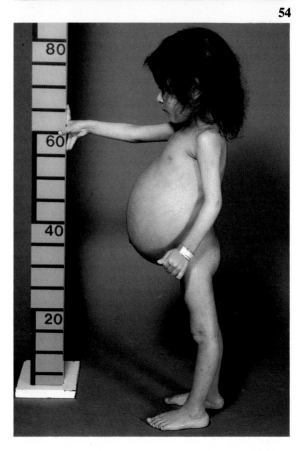

55. Ascites. This child with cirrhosis shows wasting of the chest muscles, an enlarged spleen and superficial abdominal veins due to portal hypertension. A dressing covers the site of a diagnostic tap of the peritoneal cavity. The circular white scars on the abdomen of this Arab child result from native treatment.

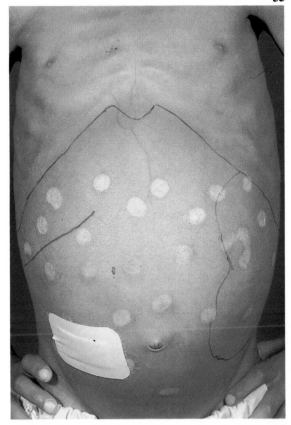

56. Peripheral oedema usually appears at the same time as ascites causing tense, shiny, swollen legs which pit on pressure as in this cirrhotic woman.

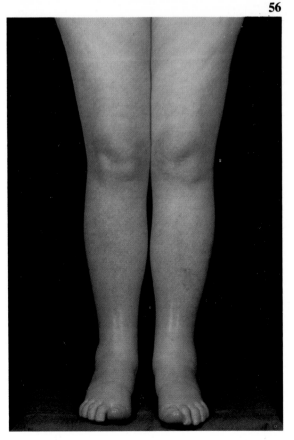

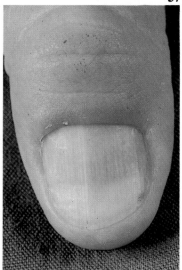

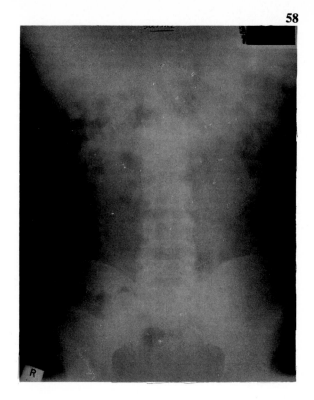

57. Hypoalbuminaemia in cirrhosis may result in these horizontal white bands across the distal part of the finger nails.

58. Abdominal x-ray in a patient with ascites shows a generalised ground glass appearance which obscures intra abdominal organs.

59. Ovarian cysts when very large may be confused with ascites. However, with an ovarian cyst the maximal dullness is in the centre of the abdomen and not in the flanks and the maximum circumference of the abdomen is below the umbilicus.

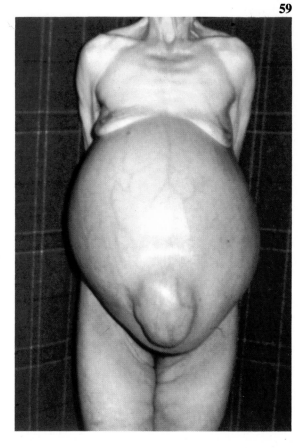

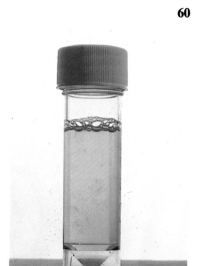
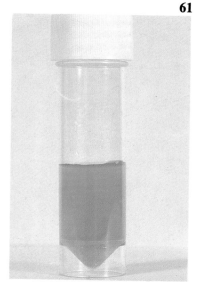
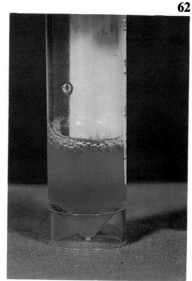

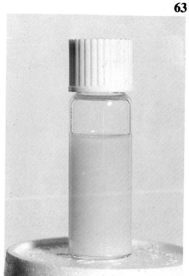

60. Ascitic fluid. A diagnostic tap (50ml) should be performed on every patient with ascites. This normally results in a clear, straw-coloured fluid with a low protein concentration (10–20g/litre) and containing up to 200 cells/mm^3 which are mainly endothelial.

61. Infected ascites. In cirrhosis occult ascitic infections are important causes of general deterioration, often with few if any abnormal signs. The fluid is usually turbid and contains over 300 cells/mm^3, mainly polymorphonuclear leucocytes. Enteric bacteria are commonly cultured, but tuberculous peritonitis must always be considered.

62. Malignant ascites is often bloodstained with a high protein concentration (above 30g/litre) and cytology may reveal malignant cells.

63. Chylous ascites is a milky fluid containing chylomicrons and is due to lymphatic obstruction, usually by a tumour. The lipid concentration of the ascites is usually twice that of plasma. Ascites containing a lower concentration of lipid (similar to plasma) is known as pseudochylous ascites and may be a complication of cirrhosis.

64. Hydrothorax. A pleural effusion is occasionally found in association with ascites. It is usually right-sided and arises by the passage of ascites through defects in the diaphragm into the pleural cavity.

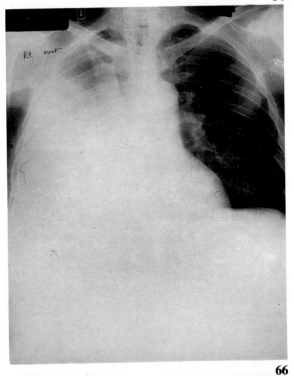

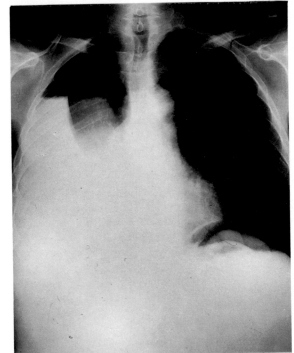

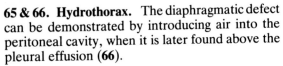

65 & 66. Hydrothorax. The diaphragmatic defect can be demonstrated by introducing air into the peritoneal cavity, when it is later found above the pleural effusion (**66**).

2. *Hepatitis*

Viral hepatitis

67. Type A virus is an RNA containing picorna virus (diameter 27nm) and can be identified by immune electron microscopy in liver and faeces. This virus causes acute hepatitis usually in children and young adults. The virus is excreted in the faeces for two weeks prior to the onset of jaundice and is spread by faecal oral contamination. When jaundiced the patient is usually no longer infectious. Type A hepatitis occurs throughout the world with the highest incidence in countries with low standards of public health.

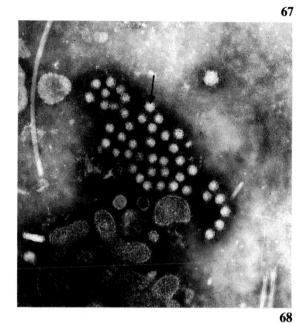

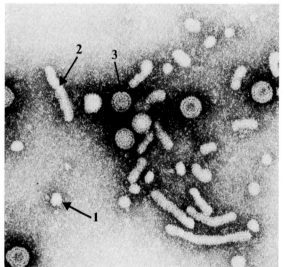

68. Type B virus is a unique DNA virus. Electron microscopy shows three components: small spheres (1, diameter 28nm), tubules (2), which are groups of small spheres, and Dane particles (3, 42nm), which are probably the infective virions. The small spheres and tubules, viral coat lipoproteins, are the hepatitis B surface antigen (HBsAg). This virus causes both acute and chronic hepatitis. Type B hepatitis is distributed throughout the world, especially prevalent in the tropics where it is a major cause of chronic liver disease (chronic hepatitis and cirrhosis) and primary liver cancer.

69. Tattooing with needles which are used repeatedly in poor hygienic conditions carries the risk of transmitting type B hepatitis. This 57-year-old man was extensively tattooed as a young man and now has decompensated cirrhosis following type B hepatitis.

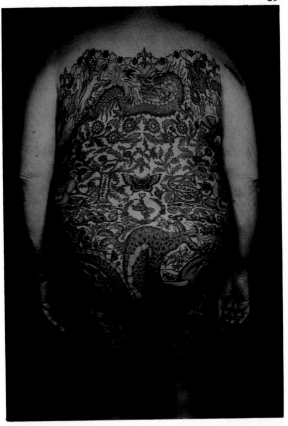

70. Drug addicts who abuse intravenous drugs often share syringes and needles which transmit type B hepatitis. The superficial thrombophlebitis in this young addict reveals the source of his acute hepatitis.

Type A and type B viruses do not account for all viral hepatitis and others (non A non B) remain to be identified. Some of these other viruses probably cause chronic liver disease.

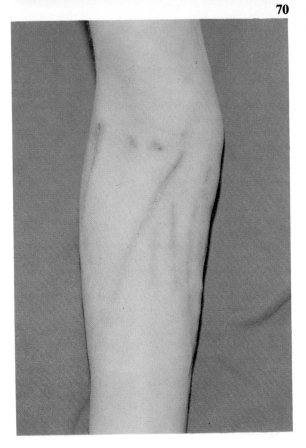

Acute viral hepatitis

71. Acute hepatitis. The clinical picture is identical in both type A and type B hepatitis. However, there is clinical hepatitis with jaundice in only a small proportion of patients infected with these viruses. Anorexia is usual a few days before the appearance of jaundice and smoking and alcohol are avoided. Malaise, nausea, vomiting and discomfort or pain under the right costal margin may be prominent. Transient rashes and arthralgia also occur. Shortly before the appearance of jaundice the urine becomes dark and the stools pale. The liver is usually slightly enlarged with a smooth tender edge. The illness lasts between two and six weeks. This patient had acute type A hepatitis (the serum bilirubin level was 16mg/100ml; 272µmol/l).

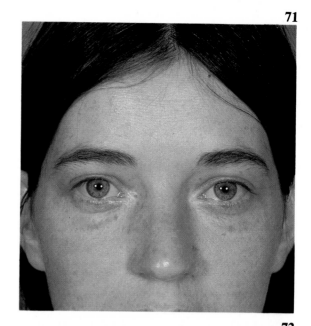

72. Thrombocytopenia is a part of the pancytopenia which occurs in viral hepatitis. Occasionally, in severe hepatitis, the thrombocytopenia is sufficient to result in generalised purpura as in this patient with type A hepatitis.

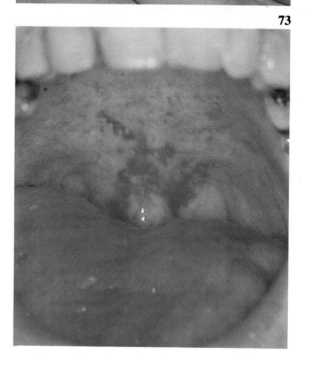

73. Purpura is also present on the palate of this patient.

74. Bruising has resulted from intramuscular injections in this patient. This reflects the clotting disorder in acute hepatitis.

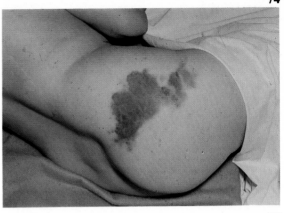

75. Vasculitis, another feature of viral hepatitis, is the cause of this rash. This allergic vasculitis is more common in type B hepatitis and may be severe, resulting in polyarteritis nodosa with glomerulonephritis and renal failure.

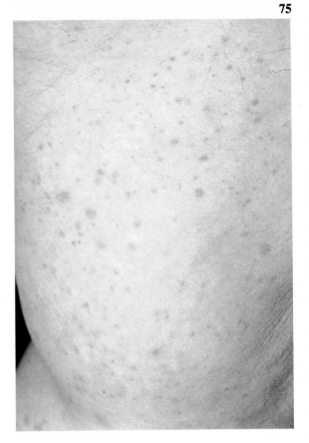

76. Liver biopsy appearances are similar in both type A and type B hepatitis. The whole liver is involved. Liver cell necrosis is most marked in the centres of the lobules. This biopsy shows a large area around the central hepatic vein (1) devoid of liver cells, only cell debris and acute inflammatory cells remain. *(H. & E. ×40)*

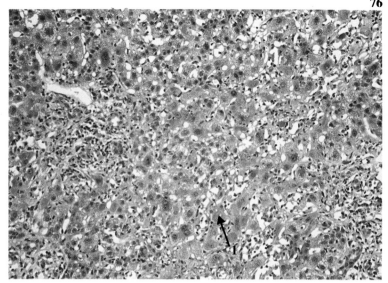

77. Liver biopsy at higher magnification shows prominent swollen cells, mitoses and eosinophilic changes in the cytoplasm of some cells (acidophilic or councilman bodies). *(H. & E. ×63)*

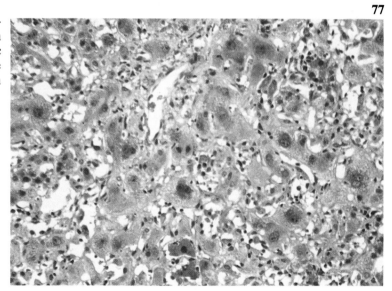

78. Portal tracts are expanded by infiltration with acute inflammatory cells, mainly leucocytes and histiocytes. Fatty infiltration is noticeably absent. The reticulin is usually well preserved and acts as a framework for the new liver cells during recovery. *(H. & E. ×50)*

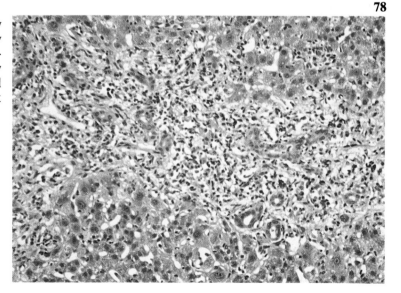

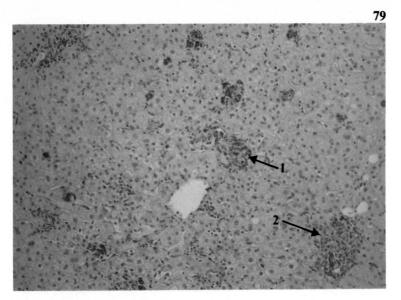

79. Resolving viral hepatitis. A biopsy late in the course of viral hepatitis shows focal areas of 'spotty' necrosis (1) scattered throughout the lobule. Mild portal tract inflammation (2) is also present. *(Diastase periodic acid Schiff×40)*

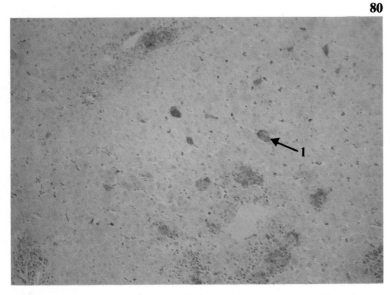

80. Resolving viral hepatitis. The biopsy shown in **79** has been stained for iron. During recovery iron is found in the Kuppfer cells (1). This reflects the increased reticulo-endothelial activity in the liver during recovery from viral hepatitis. *(Perls×40)*

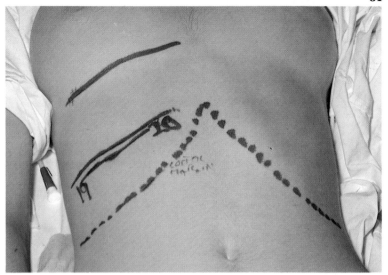

81. Fulminant hepatitis may result from both type A and type B hepatitis. This most severe form of viral hepatitis often develops suddenly, before the patient is very jaundiced. The prodroma of persistent vomiting, nightmares and confusion rapidly develop into drowsiness and coma. Prognosis is related to the depth of coma and also to liver size. The liver of this patient with fulminant type B hepatitis is typically small and daily measurement of the lower border of liver dullness by percussion shows it to be shrinking, which is a bad sign.

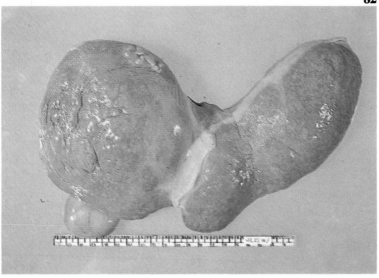

82. Liver in fulminant hepatitis is small and flaccid and the capsule is wrinkled. The left lobe is particularly shrunken.

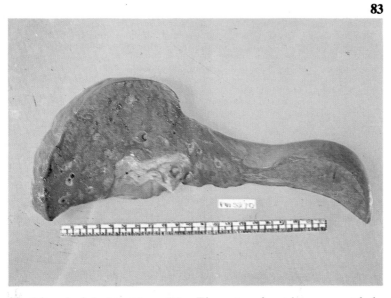

83. Liver in fulminant hepatitis. The cut surface shows a mottled appearance with yellow areas of necrosis adjacent to red areas of haemorrhage. Histologically there is massive hepatic necrosis with loss of the normal lobular structure due to collapse of the reticulin.

84. Regenerating nodules of normal liver are present in patients dying more than two weeks after the onset of acute hepatic failure due to hepatitis.

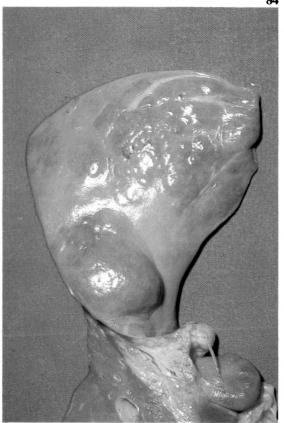

85. Cholestatic viral hepatitis is seen in some patients with acute viral hepatitis. Following the normal prodromal phase of acute viral hepatitis, a deep green-yellow jaundice and marked itching develop. The liver is enlarged. The serum bilirubin in this patient was 30mg/100ml (510μmol/l). The cholestatic phase usually disappears in two months but may last up to one year. The patient feels well. The ultimate prognosis is excellent. Cholestatic viral hepatitis must be distinguished from other causes of cholestasis, particularly extrahepatic biliary obstruction and drug related cholestasis.

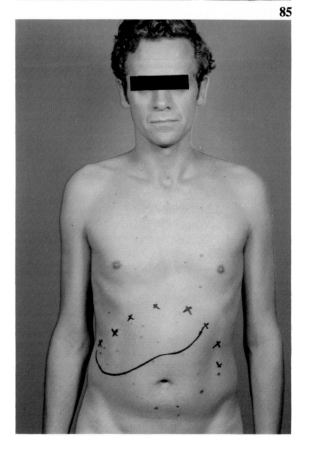

Chronic viral hepatitis

Type A hepatitis is self limiting and does not cause chronic liver disease. In contrast, type B hepatitis may pursue several courses. The virus may cause asymptomatic or symptomatic acute hepatitis and then be cleared from the body. Occasionally the patient becomes a chronic carrier of the B virus. Some carriers have histologically normal livers ('healthy carriers') while others develop chronic liver disease. Chronic type B hepatitis is commoner in males.

The pathological course of chronic type B hepatitis

This is usually assessed by liver biopsy, performed when the acute changes have subsided.

86

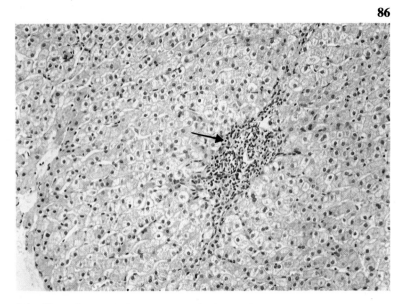

86. Chronic persistent hepatitis is found following acute hepatitis and in healthy carriers. This biopsy comes from a fit young man found to be HBsAg positive at a blood donor session. The portal tract is expanded with mononuclear cells but the limiting plate of hepatocytes is intact and there is no piecemeal necrosis of liver cells. The reticulin framework is normal. This picture may persist for years, but the prognosis is good. *(H. & E. ×50)*

87. HBsAg containing hepatocytes are present in the biopsies of chronic carriers. This biopsy is full of large cells with pale pink 'ground glass' cytoplasm. This represents a hypertrophic endoplasmic reticulum containing HBsAg. *(H. & E. ×100)*

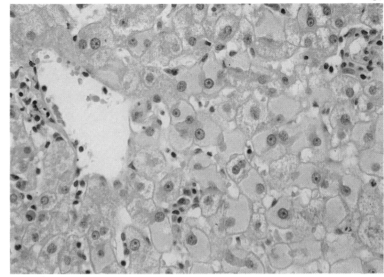

88. Orcein stain shows the liver cells containing HBsAg more clearly as groups of dark pink staining cells. *(×100)*

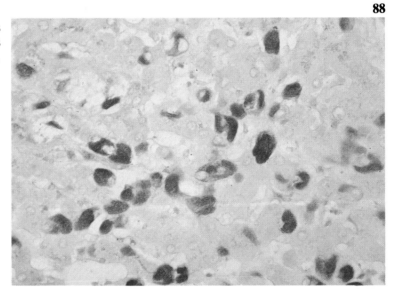

89. Peroxidase-antiperoxidase coupled with HBsAb specifically stains those cells which contain HBsAg a yellow brown colour. *(×100)*

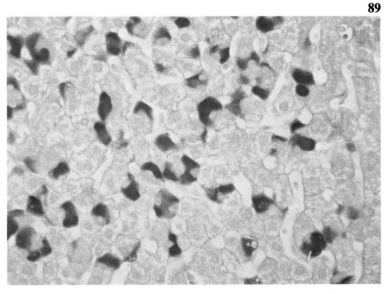

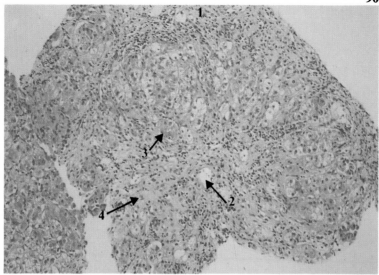

90. Chronic active hepatitis, formerly called chronic aggressive hepatitis, is the pathological description of this very active liver lesion. The portal tracts are enlarged with a heavy infiltrate of chronic inflammatory cells, mainly plasma cells and lymphocytes (1). From the portal tracts, active fibrous septa extend to the central veins (2) isolating groups of ballooned hepatocytes to form rosettes (3). The limiting plate of liver cells around the portal tract is no longer distinct but eroded by piecemeal necrosis and fibrosis. Bridging hepatic necrosis (4) has developed. *(H. & E. ×40)*

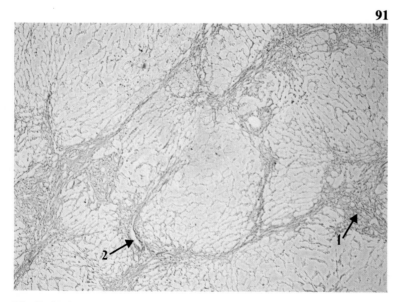

91. Bridging necrosis accompanies chronic active hepatitis, when liver cell necrosis is followed by fibrosis. The fibrosis links portal tracts (1) to hepatic veins (2) disrupting the normal lobular architecture (reticulin×24). These active fibrous septa may be the precursors of cirrhosis.

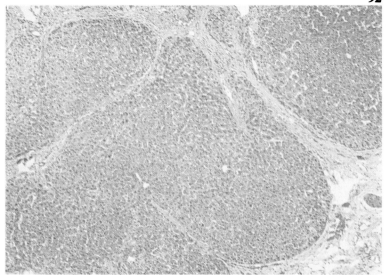

92. Inactive macronodular cirrhosis may be the end result of chronic active hepatitis due to type B hepatitis. Following extensive liver cell necrosis and reticulin collapse, some liver cells regenerate to form nodules of various sizes separated by septa of inactive fibrous tissue. The normal lobular architecture of the liver is lost. *(H.&E.×10)*

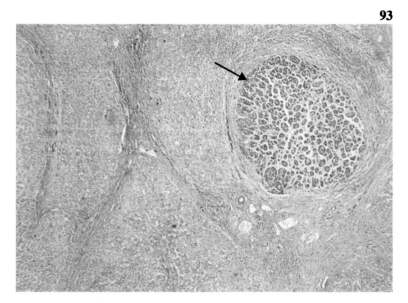

93. Primary liver cancer is the final complication of chronic type B hepatitis. It is usually seen in patients with established cirrhosis and is often heralded by sudden deterioration of liver cell function and ascites. In many patients α fetoprotein appears in the blood. Occasionally, a small primary liver cancer is an incidental finding at autopsy as in this patient with inactive cirrhosis who died from liver failure. *(Martius-Scarlet-Blue ×10)*

94. Peritoneoscopy is valuable in chronic hepatitis to establish whether cirrhosis is present. The transition of chronic active hepatitis to cirrhosis may not be visible in a small liver biopsy specimen. However the nodularity of the liver surface characteristic of cirrhosis is easily seen at peritoneoscopy. In this patient, who is HBsAg positive, the shrunken, nodular liver clearly indicates cirrhosis.

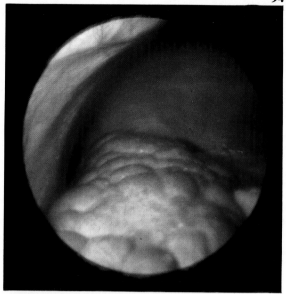

95. Decompensated cirrhosis with portal hypertension and ascites eventually develops in many patients with cirrhosis due to type B hepatitis. This cirrhotic patient first presented when ascites appeared. The dressing covers the site of a diagnostic peritoneal tap performed to exclude ascitic infection.

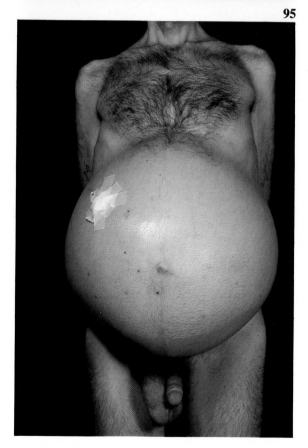

Lupoid hepatitis
(non B chronic active hepatitis)

This chronic hepatitis affects women predominantly (75%), usually young adults but also women around the menopause. The aetiology is unknown and tests for HBsAg are always negative. Immunological changes include the presence in the blood of anti-nuclear factor in about 50% of cases, smooth muscle antibody in about 66%, and a very high serum gammaglobulin (particularly the IgG fraction). Other diseases are frequently associated, including diabetes mellitus, thyroiditis, fibrosing alveolitis, pericarditis and myocarditis, renal tubular acidosis, ulcerative colitis, autoimmune haemolytic anaemia and vasculitis. The illness may start as acute viral hepatitis. However, the onset is usually insidious with a mild fluctuating jaundice, fevers, malaise and tiredness. Untreated, lupoid hepatitis progresses to cirrhosis. Portal hypertension and portal systemic encephalopathy are late features. Spider naevi are usually present and moderate hepato-splenomegaly is usual.

96. Acne vulgaris and a moon shaped facies are common at the presentation of lupoid hepatitis, even before prednisolone treatment.

97. Striae develop on the abdomen, buttocks, thighs and upper arms. This sign together with the acne and a moon face sometimes lead to lupoid hepatitis being confused with Cushing's syndrome.

96

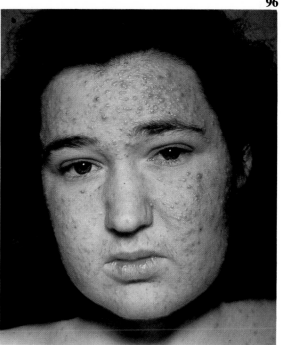

97

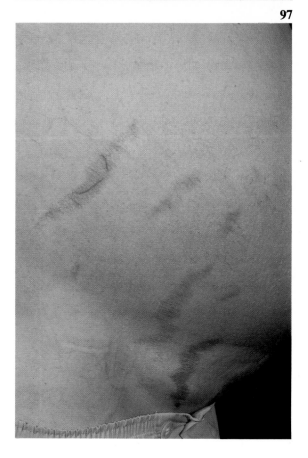

98. Bruising around injection and venepuncture sites in this patient with lupoid hepatitis is due to a clotting disorder which may be severe. The prothrombin time is prolonged and there is thrombocytopenia.

99. Purpura results when the thrombocytopenia is profound in lupoid hepatitis.

100. Butterfly rash may be seen in non B (lupoid) chronic active hepatitis. This erythematous rash on the cheeks and the bridge of the nose is similar to that seen in systemic lupus erythematosus. Despite the occasional finding of L.E. cells in the blood (in about 15% of patients), the full syndrome of systemic lupus erythematosus does not occur.

101. Vitiligo is shown as patchy depigmentation and hyperpigmentation and is present in some patients with lupoid hepatitis.

102. Splinter haemorrhages in the nails of this patient with lupoid hepatitis are a sign of a widespread vasculitis.

103. Vasculitis has resulted in these dark pin head lesions on the hand of a patient with lupoid hepatitis. Later, the lesions may undergo necrosis and ulcerate.

104. Erythema nodosum-like rash is also the result of vasculitis in this patient. The blotchy erythematous areas are slightly raised and painful.

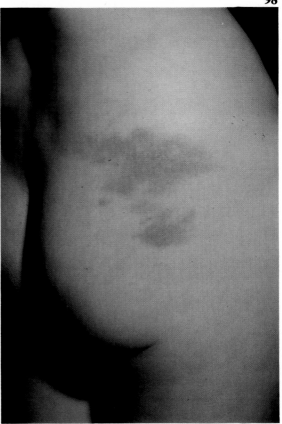

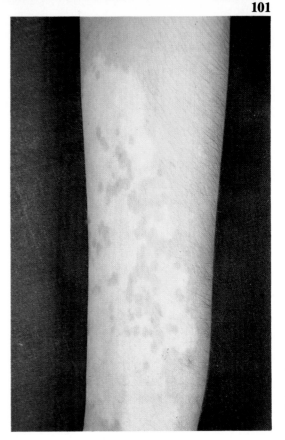

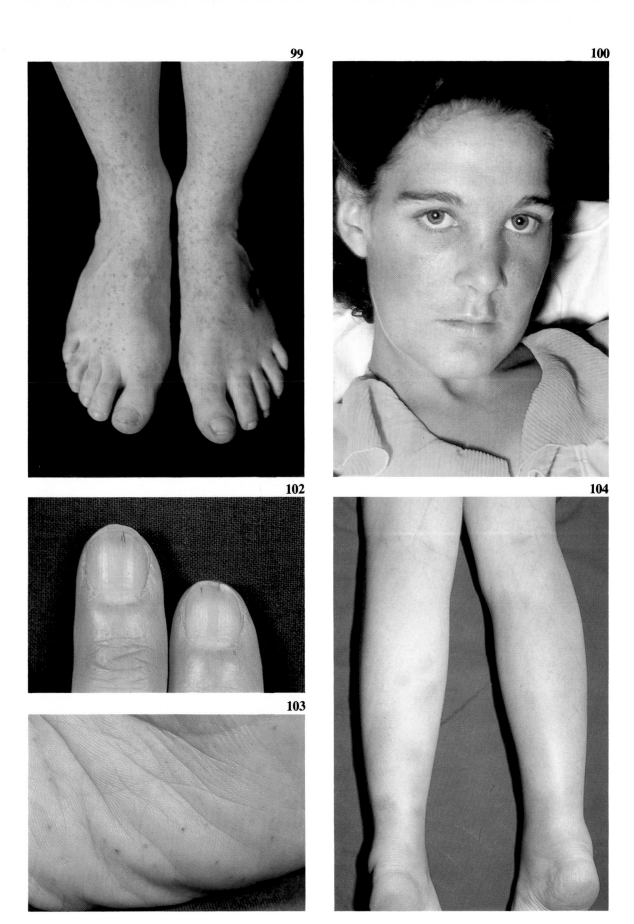

105–107. Superficial gangrene may rarely follow a severe vasculitis. The progression of the lesion over two weeks, despite high dose predniso-lone therapy, can be seen in this patient with lupoid hepatitis. Linear red vasculitic lesions of her right foot rapidly led to infarction of a large area of skin.

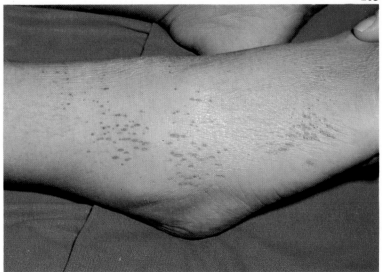

106. The white infarcted area became clearly demarcated from the surrounding erythematous skin.

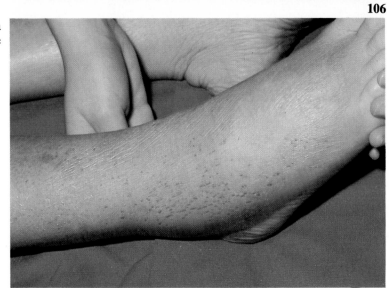

107. Necrosis of this area was fol-lowed by sloughing of the skin to reveal the underlying tendons.

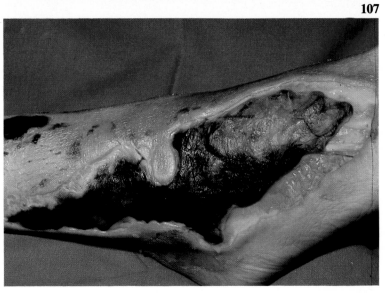

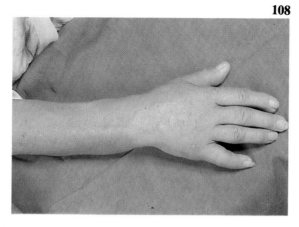

108. Arthritis affecting the larger joints, such as the wrist and elbow is common. Occasionally an arthritis with all the features of acute rheumatoid arthritis may develop as in this patient with boggy swelling of the wrist and proximal interphalangeal joints.

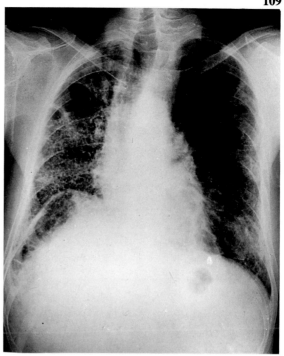

109. Fibrosing alveolitis. Occasionally, frank fibrosing alveolitis develops. This man's lupoid hepatitis has been inactive for several years as a result of prednisolone therapy. However he has severe exertional dyspnoea and the chest x-ray shows a honeycomb lung with bullae.

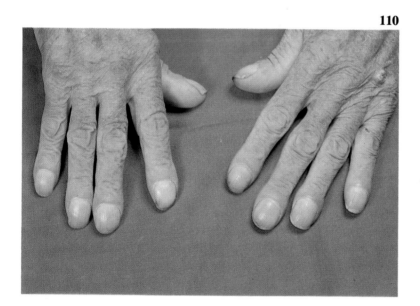

110. Finger clubbing is severe in the presence of fibrosing alveolitis. These spade-like fingers are from the patient shown in **109**.

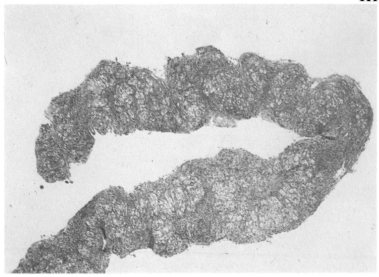

111. Liver biopsy in non B chronic active hepatitis usually shows florid changes with infiltration of chronic inflammatory cells expanding the portal tracts and spilling out into the lobule. Liver cell necrosis and rosette formation may be so prominent that they can be seen at low magnification. *(H. & E. ×10)*

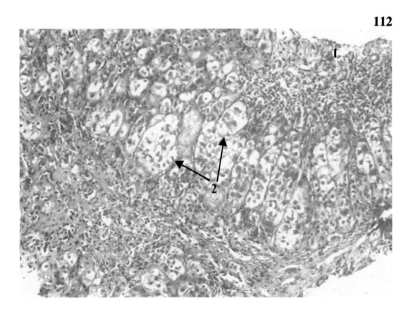

112. Liver biopsy. At a higher magnification the activity of the chronic hepatitis is obvious. Active fibrous septa extend from the enlarged portal tract (1) towards the central vein enclosing groups of dilated and degenerating liver cells to form rosettes (2). The limiting plate of the portal tract has disappeared as a result of piecemeal necrosis of liver cells and fibrosis. This histological picture is identical to the chronic active hepatitis caused by type B hepatitis. These conditions cannot usually be distinguished on histological grounds using routine stains. *(H. & E. ×40)*

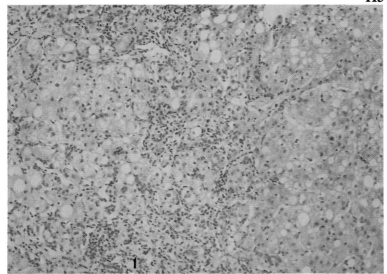

113. Chronic active hepatitis. In a milder case the portal tract (1) is expanded by infiltration with chronic inflammatory cells. Active fibrous septa extend into the lobule. There is piecemeal necrosis of the limiting plate of liver cells around the portal tract and some fatty infiltration. *(H. & E. ×40)*

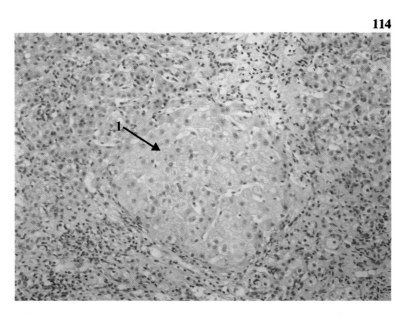

114. Chronic active hepatitis. As the liver cell necrosis and fibrosis progress regenerative nodules of liver cells develop. This biopsy has included a small regenerative nodule (1) in the midst of an area of active liver cell destruction. *(H. & E. ×40)*

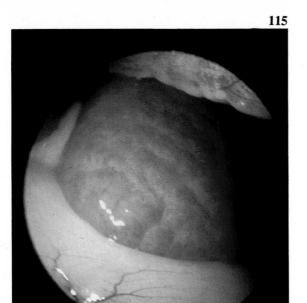

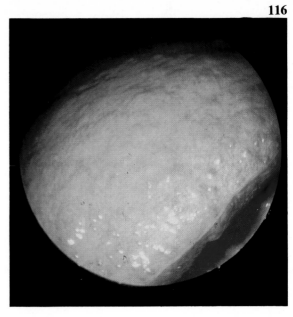

115. Peritoneoscopy is employed to determine whether lupoid hepatitis has progressed to cirrhosis. The liver biopsy may be insufficient due to the sampling error with a small specimen. The lobulated appearance of the liver in this patient with lupoid hepatitis indicates a non-cirrhotic liver.

116. Peritoneoscopy in this patient with lupoid hepatitis shows a uniformly nodular liver surface indicating cirrhosis.

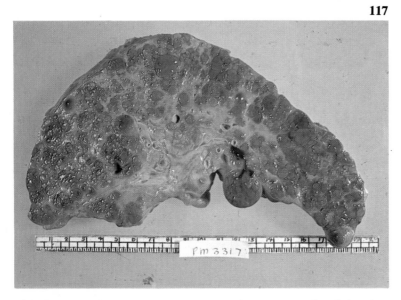

117. Macronodular cirrhosis may be the end result of lupoid hepatitis. As the disease progresses inflammatory infiltration of the liver decreases and wide fibrous bands, separating nodules of varying sizes, are seen. At autopsy an inactive cirrhosis may be found.

Drug-induced hepatitis

Drugs may cause both acute and chronic hepatitis. Drug-induced hepatitis is often more severe in patients who are also receiving drugs which induce hepatic microsomal enzymes, such as phenobarbitone or alcohol. Liver histology in drug-induced hepatitis is usually indistinguishable from viral hepatitis except that liver cell necrosis may be more extensive.

Acute drug-induced hepatitis

118. Paracetamol (acetominophen) hepatitis usually results from intentional overdosage. Following ingestion, nausea and vomiting occur. The symptoms then subside for one or two days when mild jaundice and liver tenderness appear. As little as 7.5g (15 tablets) may cause hepatitis and 25g (50 tablets) have been fatal. In severe cases, such as this patient, who had consumed over 100 tablets, drowsiness and coma rapidly develop. Death occurs between the 4th and 18th day. The prothrombin time is prolonged.

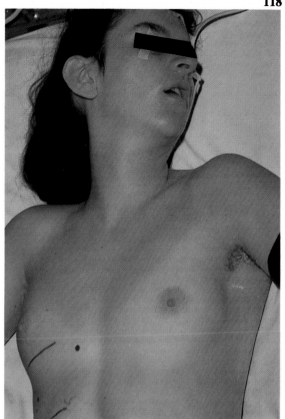

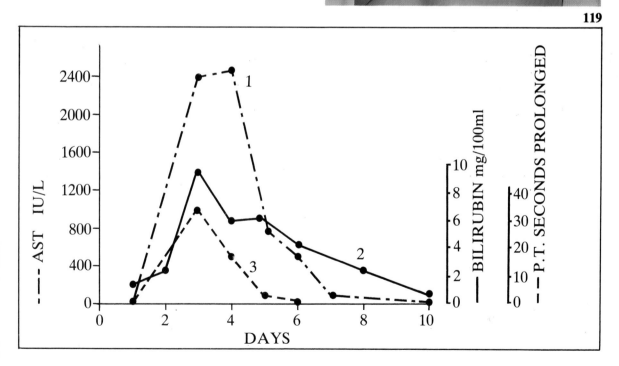

119. Paracetamol hepatitis. This 27-year-old man took an overdose of 130 tablets (65g) of paracetamol and recovered. Three days after the overdose the serum aspartate transaminase (SGOT) concentration (1) had risen to 2400 iu/litre and the bilirubin level (2) was 5mg/100ml (85 µmol/l). The prothrombin time (3) was prolonged 40 seconds over the control time. Despite this massive hepatitis, all the tests had returned to normal 10 days after the overdose.

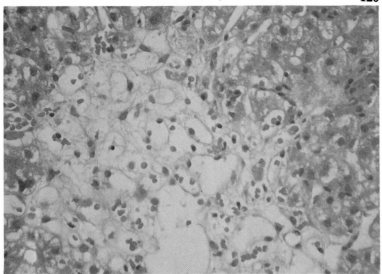

120. Paracetamol hepatitis. The liver biopsy shows well demarcated centrizonal necrosis of liver cells and collapse of the reticulin framework. In surviving patients the liver lesion heals completely apart from some residual central fibrosis. *(H. & E. ×100)*

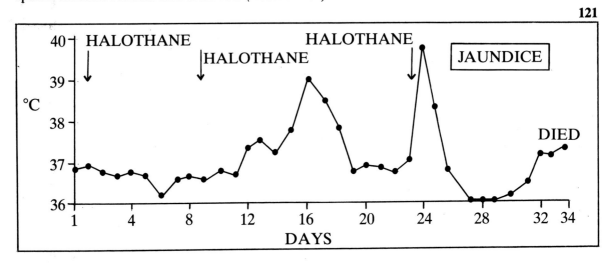

121. Halothane hepatitis is uncommon. It usually follows repeated anaesthetics, often for minor surgical procedures. A history of unexplained fevers five to seven days after a previous halothane exposure is often obtained. Following a subsequent halothane anaesthetic, a moderate to high fever develops early (one to three days) occasionally with a rash and arthralgia. Jaundice appears three to four days later and rapidly deepens. Anorexia, nausea and vomiting may be prominent. The onset of drowsiness and coma indicate a poor prognosis. This patient had three halothane anaesthetics. There was no fever after the first anaesthetic. Six days after the second halothane exposure a pyrexia developed and reached a peak of 39°C. One day after the third anaesthetic he had a fever of 39.5°C and three days later he was jaundiced. The patient died 11 days after the third halothane anaesthetic.

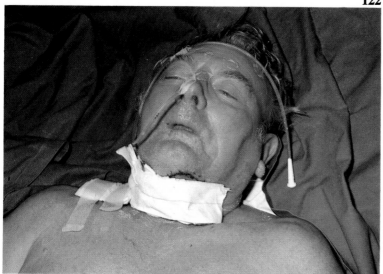

122. Halothane hepatitis in this 72-year-old man, with carcinoma of the tongue, has followed three halothane anaesthetics for tumour biopsy and for a block dissection of the neck. His temperature chart is shown in **121**. He is obese, jaundiced and in hepatic coma. Obese patients tend to have a poor prognosis. The patient died two days later. Although clinical halothane hepatitis is uncommon, minor disturbances of liver function follow about 10% of halothane anaesthetics.

123

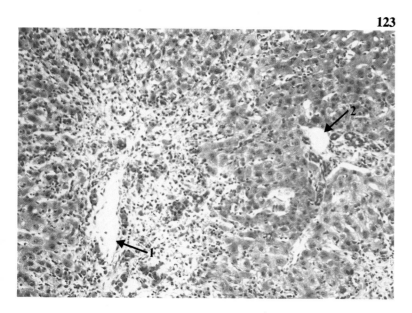

123. Halothane hepatitis. The liver biopsy shows similar changes to viral hepatitis although they are usually more severe. Extensive necrosis and haemorrhage is present around the hepatic vein (1) but the portal tracts (2) are spared. *(H. & E. ×40)*

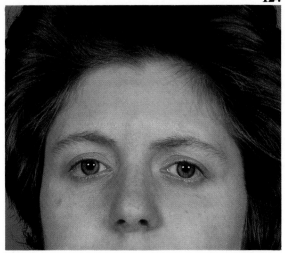

124. Isoniazid hepatitis. Clinical isoniazid hepatitis is uncommon but severe. The patients are usually over 35 years old and have taken isoniazid for three to four months when malaise, lassitude, anorexia and fevers herald the onset of hepatitis. Jaundice with hepatomegaly follows in two to four weeks. The jaundice may be prolonged, even after stopping the drug. This patient had taken isoniazid and rifampicin for six months when jaundice appeared. She was jaundiced with a severe hepatitis for five weeks. Death from acute hepatic failure can occur. This patient recovered.

125

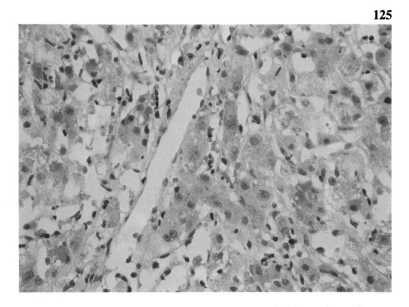

125. Isoniazid hepatitis. The liver biopsy of this patient shows extensive centrizonal necrosis, acute inflammatory infiltration and haemorrhage. In most patients who survive the liver recovers completely. Rarely, isoniazid may cause chronic active hepatitis which develops insidiously without preceding acute hepatitis. *(H. & E. ×100)*

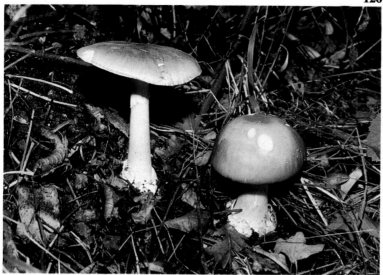

126. Amanita phalloides is the only mushroom known to be hepatotoxic to man. Ingestion causes fulminant hepatic failure, usually in the autumn among holiday-makers who are unfamiliar with the recognition of edible fungi. Amanita phalloides is distinguished by a pale yellow to olive green cap and crowded white gills. The stipe (stem) has a bulbous base and is white, but may have a greenish tinge. Symptoms are delayed for 6 to 15 hours after poisoning with Amanita phalloides. Nausea, vomiting, abdominal cramps and diarrhoea are followed by signs of dehydration and vasomotor collapse. Jaundice and hepatic coma appear after three days. Signs of renal and central nervous system damage are also prominent.

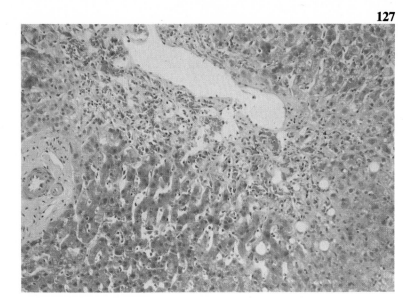

127. Amanita phalloides. The liver biopsy shows massive centri-lobular liver cell necrosis, infiltration with acute inflammatory cells and haemorrhage. Many liver cells contain fat droplets. *(H & E. × 40)*

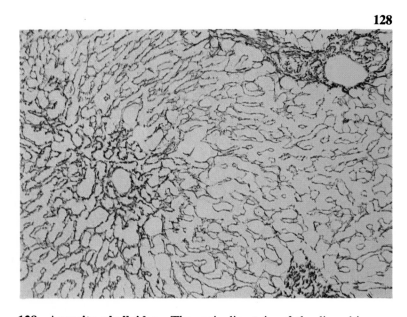

128. Amanita phalloides. The reticulin stain of the liver biopsy shows more clearly the collapse of the reticulin framework around the central veins. *(× 40)*

Chronic drug-induced hepatitis

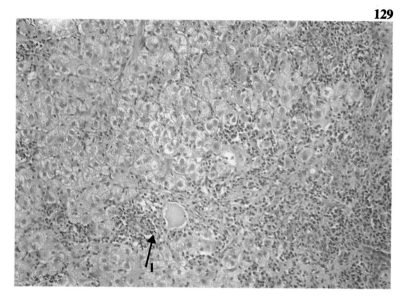

129. Oxyphenisatin is one of several drugs which can result in chronic active hepatitis indistinguishable from lupoid hepatitis. Liver damage usually appears after at least a year of regular use of this laxative. The liver biopsy changes are similar to those of lupoid hepatitis. The portal zones (1) are infiltrated with mononuclear cells and there is piecemeal necrosis and active fibrosis. The fibrous septa extend to the centres of the lobules. In some patients the changes reverse on stopping the drug, but in others the hepatitis progresses to cirrhosis. Other drugs that may cause chronic active hepatitis are *methyl dopa* and *isoniazid* and very rarely *aspirin. (H. & E. ×40)*

Hepatitis in childhood

130. Giant cell hepatitis is the common reaction of the liver in infancy to a variety of insults. These include: infections by type B hepatitis, cytomegalovirus, herpes simplex, congenital rubella, coxsackie B and syphilis, metabolic disorders such as galactosaemia and α_1 antitrypsin deficiency and cholestatic syndromes such as biliary atresia. In about 50% of the patients no cause can be found and these are termed *neonatal hepatitis*. Some of the infants are stillborn or die soon after birth, but more commonly a fluctuant cholestatic jaundice appears in the first two weeks. Jaundice has always appeared by two months. The liver and spleen are enlarged and the urine dark and faeces pale. This four-month-old infant had been jaundiced since two weeks old. No cause for her giant cell hepatitis was found. The prognosis is usually poor.

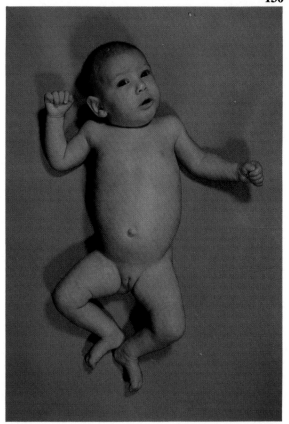

131. Giant cell hepatitis. The liver biopsy is characterised by many multinucleated giant cells, up to 400μ in diameter, scattered throughout the lobule. The portal tracts are infiltrated with inflammatory cells and there is liver cell swelling and necrosis. Centrilobular cholestasis is often prominent. *(H. & E. ×64)*

3. Cirrhosis

Cirrhosis is defined as widespread fibrosis with nodule formation.
Cirrhosis is the result of prolonged liver cell necrosis followed by
fibrosis throughout the liver. Liver fibrosis alone is not sufficient
for the diagnosis of cirrhosis, as in congenital hepatic fibrosis where
there is extensive periportal fibrosis but nodules are not present.
Conversely, the presence of liver nodules without fibrosis is not
cirrhosis. This is seen in the rare condition partial nodular transformation. Cirrhosis may be the end result of many liver diseases
including chronic viral hepatitis, non B chronic active hepatitis,
alcoholism, chronic biliary obstruction, haemochromatosis, Wilson's
disease, heart failure and hepatic venous obstruction, α_1 antitrypsin
deficiency and drug toxicity (such as oxyphenisatin and methotrexate).
During the development of cirrhosis different patterns of fibrosis
may help to distinguish between the different causes. In haemochromatosis the fibrous septa radiate from the portal tracts to give
a pointed pattern resembling a holly leaf. In biliary obstruction the
fibrosis is mainly in and around the portal tracts and then spreads
out to the centres of the lobules. In heart failure fibrosis is most
marked in the centrizonal areas. Late in the course of cirrhosis liver
cell necrosis and inflammation disappear and the fibrous septa
become inactive and dense, separating regenerating nodules of
various sizes. It is then often impossible to identify the cause of
the cirrhosis. In a proportion of cirrhotic patients no cause for the
cirrhosis can be found and these are termed *cryptogenic cirrhosis*.
The regenerating nodules disrupt the flow of blood through the
liver. Obstruction to portal venous blood flow results in portal
hypertension. Shunting of blood through sinusoids at the periphery
of the nodules impairs perfusion of the nodules.

Pathological classification

Three types of cirrhosis are recognized, classified according to the size of the regenerating liver cell nodules.

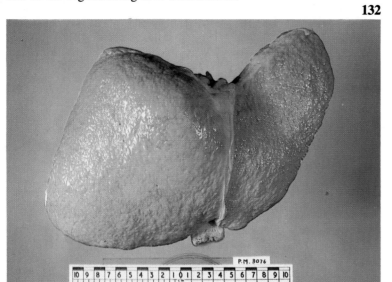

132

132. Micronodular cirrhosis consists of small regenerating nodules of approximately equal size separated by regular bands of fibrous tissue. Every lobule is involved. This type of cirrhosis is usually associated with a continuing liver insult such as alcohol.

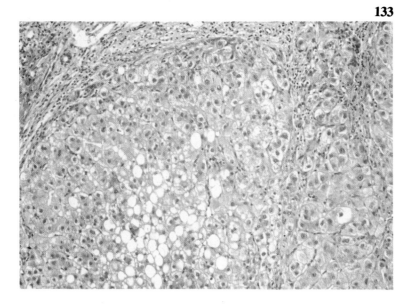

133

133. Micronodular cirrhosis. The liver biopsy shows fibrous septa enclosing small nodules of liver cells. Many of the hepatocytes are necrotic and there is marked fatty infiltration. This biopsy comes from a patient with alcoholic cirrhosis. *(H. & E. ×40)*

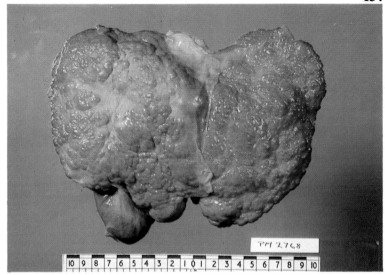

134. Macronodular cirrhosis. The liver is very misshapen and contains nodules of varying sizes. Some of the nodules are large. They are separated by irregular bands of fibrous tissue. In some of the larger nodules areas with a normal lobular architecture may be found. If a small liver biopsy sample only contains these normal lobules the presence of a macronodular cirrhosis may be missed. This cirrhosis resulted from chronic type B hepatitis.

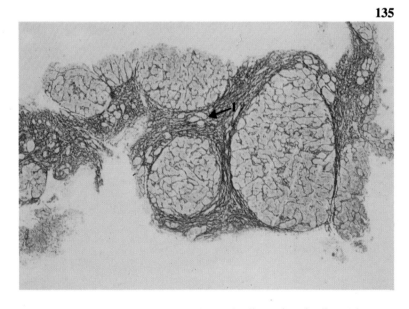

135. Macronodular cirrhosis. The reticulin stain of a liver biopsy shows clearly the variable sizes of the nodules and fibrous septa. Previous necrosis and lobular collapse have resulted in the concentration of several portal tracts (1) in the broad fibrous scars. *(×13)*

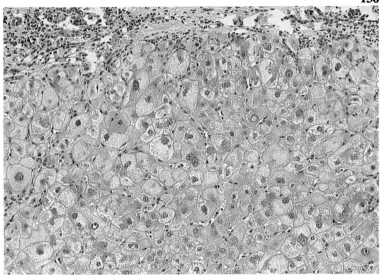

136. Macronodular cirrhosis. Regeneration in cirrhotic nodules often results in liver cell dysplasia. The hepatocytes are of different sizes and many contain large nuclei. Some liver cells are binucleate. The liver cell plates are of varying thickness. A fibrous septum enclosing this nodule is visible at the top of the picture. The liver cell dysplasia in cirrhosis may predispose to the development of primary liver cancer. *(H.&E.×100)*

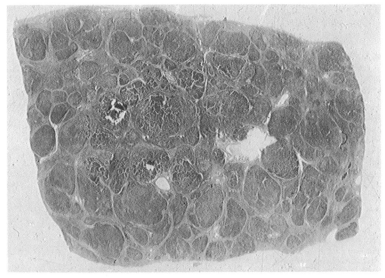

137. Mixed cirrhosis has features of both micronodular and macronodular cirrhosis. Micronodular cirrhosis may develop into a macronodular cirrhosis when the cause of the liver injury is removed. This is seen in alcoholic cirrhotics who stop drinking. A mixed cirrhosis is an intermediate stage.

Clinical signs of cirrhosis

The signs of cirrhosis stem principally from two main causes, portal hypertension and liver cell failure. These signs include spider naevi, paper money skin, palmar erythema, white nails, finger clubbing, endocrine changes such as gynaecomastia and reduced body hair in males and fluid retention with ascites and ankle oedema (see Chapter 1). Occasionally signs of the cause of the cirrhosis may be found, such as Kayser-Fleischer rings in the eyes of patients with Wilson's disease. Patients with cirrhosis are classified according to whether the condition is *compensated*, when the patient is relatively well or *decompensated*, when fluid retention and liver failure are present. Finally, other conditions are associated with cirrhosis, irrespective of the cause.

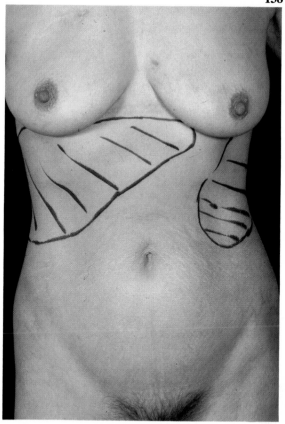

138. Splenomegaly is common in cirrhosis and usually indicates portal hypertension. In this patient with alcoholic cirrhosis the liver is also enlarged due to fatty infiltration. However there are no complications and she feels well. This is an example of a well compensated cirrhosis.

139. Abdominal wall veins in this patient with alcoholic cirrhosis are portal systemic venous collaterals and indicate portal hypertension. The direction of blood flow in these veins is away from the umbilicus. Note the presence of ascites, gynaecomastia and the scanty body hair.

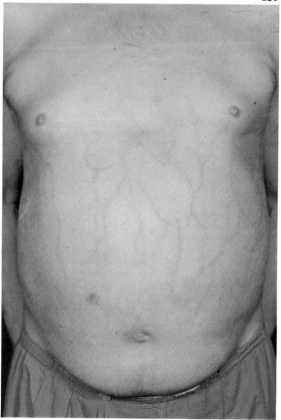

140. Abdominal herniae are common in cirrhotic patients, even in the absence of ascites. This patient has cirrhosis and ascites from chronic hepatic venous outflow obstruction (Budd-Chiari syndrome). The umbilicus has herniated and another hernia has developed through the rectus sheath. There is scanty body hair.

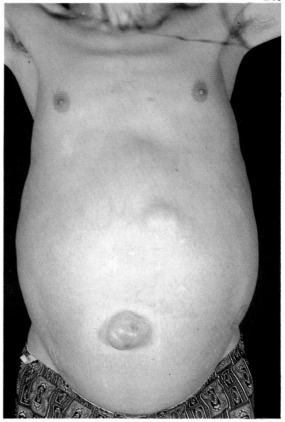

141. Gallstones are present in about 30% of cirrhotic patients compared to about 13% in a matched population. They are usually pigment stones. This endoscopic retrograde cholangiogram from a patient with chronic active hepatitis and cirrhosis has demonstrated three stones in the gall bladder.

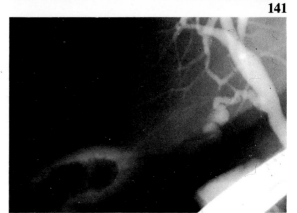

142. Recurrent haemorrhage in cirrhosis is due to failure of hepatic synthesis of clotting factors. This is a sign of liver failure and decompensated cirrhosis. This patient with alcoholic cirrhosis developed extensive bruising following a percutaneous needle liver biopsy.

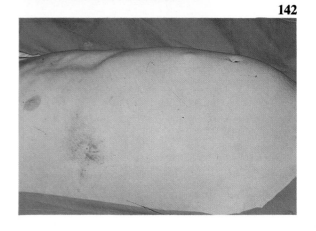

143. Decompensated cirrhosis often presents with ascites and peripheral oedema. Acites developed in this Arab patient following a haematemesis from oesophageal varices. He had cirrhosis following type B hepatitis. The liver was shrunken and the spleen was impalpable.

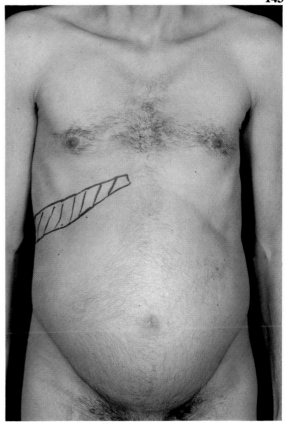

144. Decompensated cirrhosis. Deepening jaundice indicates progressive liver failure. This is usually a late sign in cirrhosis and purpura and bruising are often associated. This patient had decompensated cryptogenic cirrhosis.

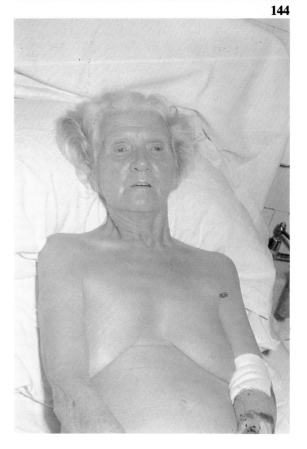

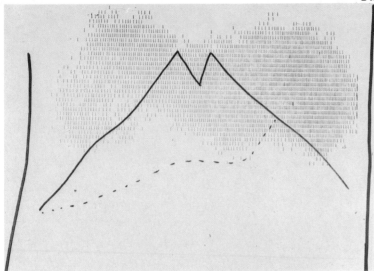

145. Isotope scan in cirrhosis shows reduced liver uptake and increased splenic uptake of ^{99}technetium. In many patients the nodularity of the cirrhotic liver results in a patchy uptake of the isotope which may be mistaken for space occupying lesions. In advanced cirrhosis very little isotope is taken up by the liver and most is seen in the spleen, as in this patient with cryptogenic cirrhosis.

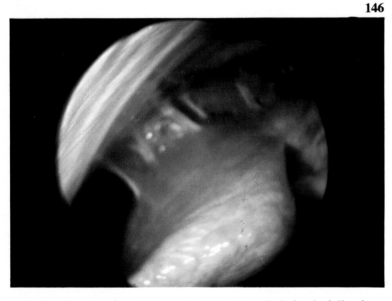

146. Peritoneoscopy. This patient developed cirrhosis following viral hepatitis. The liver is small and nodular. The adhesions between the liver capsule and the abdominal wall result from inflammation of the liver during acute viral hepatitis. Peritoneoscopy also permits biopsy of suspicious areas such as nodules of primary liver cancer which may develop in cirrhosis.

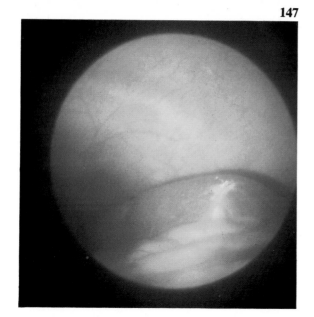

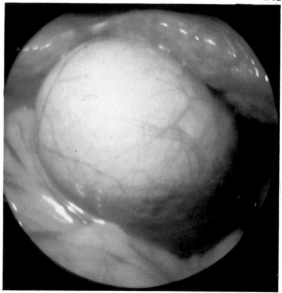

147. Peritoneoscopy. A normal spleen is not usually visible. In this patient with cryptogenic cirrhosis the spleen is clearly seen and therefore enlarged indicating the presence of portal hypertension.

148. Peritoneoscopy. This enlarged gall bladder is a normal appearance in cirrhosis and does not indicate biliary obstruction. Note the normal reddish-pink colour of the cirrhotic liver in this patient with cryptogenic cirrhosis.

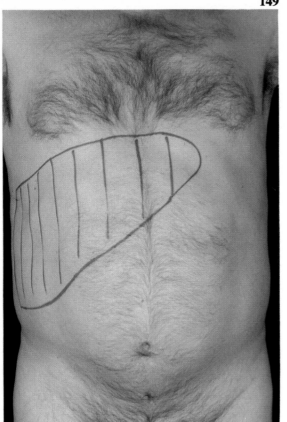

Alcoholic liver disease – clinical signs

149. Fatty liver. Hepatomegaly due to a fatty liver is an early sign of alcoholic liver disease. The liver is usually tender. On withdrawal of alcohol, fatty infiltration disappears and the liver returns to a normal size.

150. Acute alcoholic hepatitis is the next stage of alcoholic liver disease. It usually follows a particularly heavy drinking bout. Deep jaundice, as in this patient, is a bad sign. Note the prominent spider naevus on this patient's nose and her raw red tongue. The liver is usually enlarged, due to fatty infiltration in addition to the hepatitis.

151. Acute alcoholic hepatitis. These patients often have a persistent fever and a polymorph leucocytosis. Alcoholic hepatitis may be confused with acute viral hepatitis. However, the florid spider naevi of the alcoholic, seen on the chest of this patient, a large liver and a leucocytosis are not found in viral hepatitis.

150

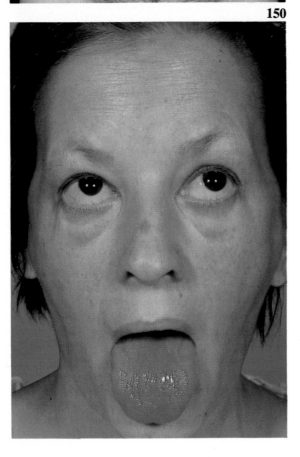

151

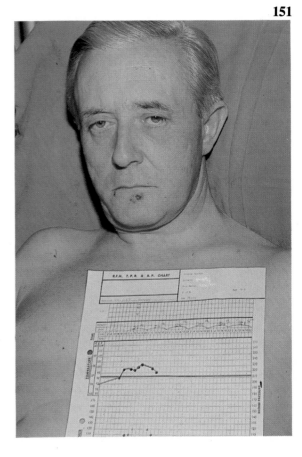

152. Isotope scan. In severe alcoholic hepatitis uptake of ^{99}technetium by the liver may be negligible. Only splenic uptake is seen.

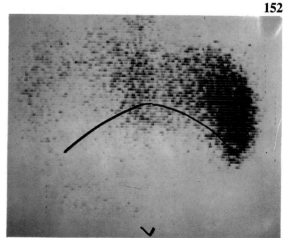

153. Decompensated alcoholic cirrhosis is the final stage of alcoholic liver disease. Note the tense ascites and scanty body hair. In contrast to acute alcoholic hepatitis, jaundice is usually absent.

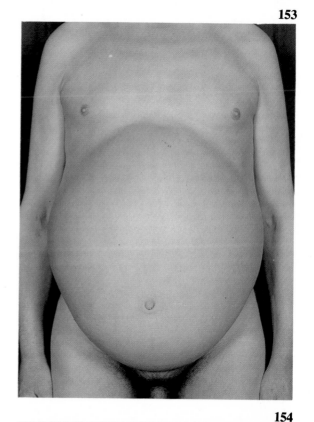

154. Spider naevi are usual and often florid. The shoulder of this alcoholic patient is covered with spider naevi.

155. Parotid enlargement occasionally occurs in alcoholic liver disease. The swelling is bilateral and painless.

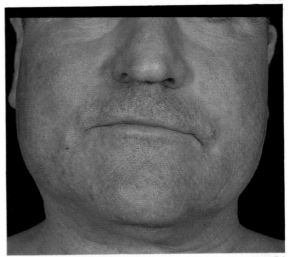

156. Dupuytren's contracture. This progressive fibrosis of the palmar fascia may cause fixed flexion deformities of the fingers. Dupuytren's contracture is more common is alcoholics than in a control population. It is especially frequent among alcoholic cirrhotics but is related to the alcoholism and not to the cirrhosis. Dupuytren's contracture may also be familial.

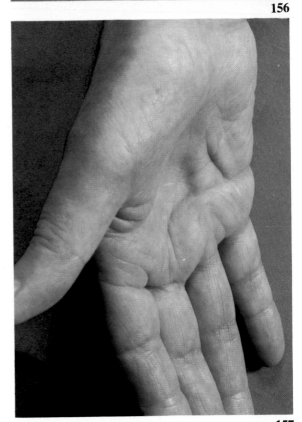

157. Red tongue is due to poor nutrition and vitamin deficiency in alcoholics. The tongue is sore and smooth due to the disappearance of the papillae. This patient also has angular cheilosis and paper money skin.

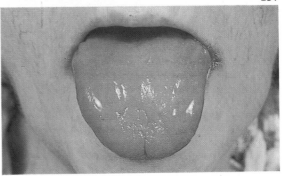

158. Alcoholic neuropathy occasionally develops in poorly nourished alcoholics. Paraesthesiae, impaired pin prick and light touch sensation and absent ankle jerks are early signs of this peripheral neuropathy. In severe cases, such as this woman, gross muscle wasting results. The calf muscles are especially wasted.

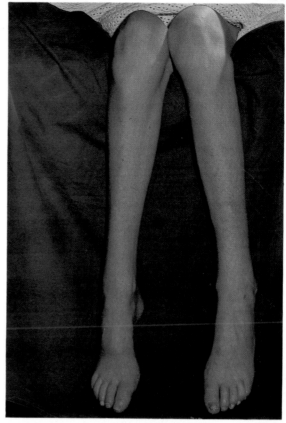

159. Beri-beri, a rare complication of alcoholism develops when malnutrition has resulted in gross thiamine deficiency. The 'wet' beri-beri syndrome presents as severe congestive cardiac failure which responds dramatically to thiamine. This patient has pitting oedema up to his chest.

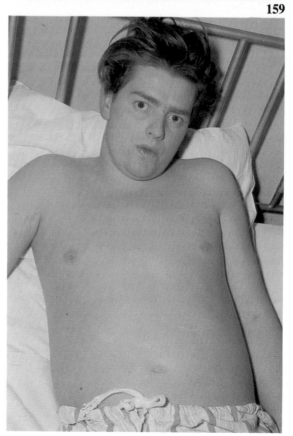

160. Bruising, which may be extensive, is common in alcoholics and usually due to repeated falls while drunk. This patient had alcoholic cirrhosis.

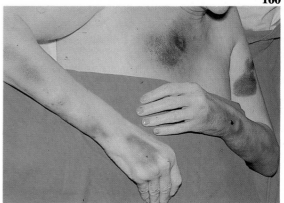

161. Bruising around the eye of this woman with alcoholic cirrhosis followed a fight.

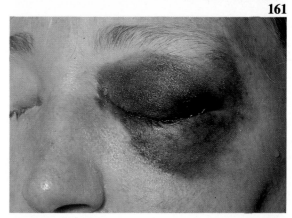

162. Acne rosacea is more common in middle aged alcoholics than in a control population. This acneiform rash affects principally the malar prominences, nose, forehead and chin. This patient had alcoholic cirrhosis.

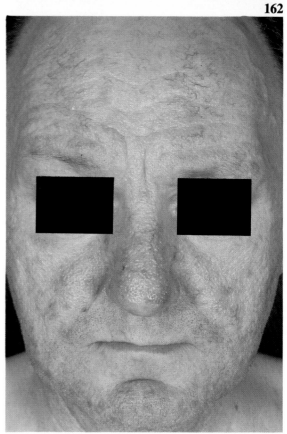

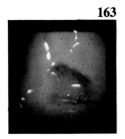

163. Duodenal ulcer. The incidence of duodenal ulcer is higher in alcoholic cirrhosis than in other forms of cirrhosis. This endoscopic picture from an alcoholic shows a large duodenal ulcer covered by a pale slough.

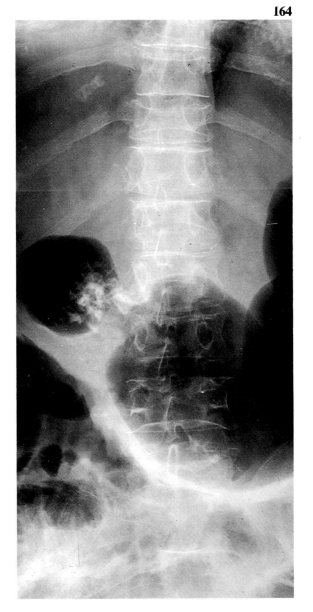

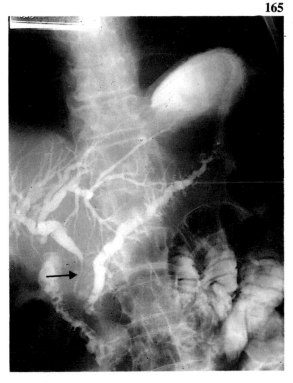

165. Chronic calcific pancreatitis in alcoholics occasionally causes a biliary stricture resulting in cholestatic (obstructive type) jaundice. The endoscopic retrograde cholangiopancreatogram in this alcoholic woman showed a dilated pancreatic duct and dilated side branches. These changes suggest chronic pancreatitis. A long stricture (arrow) of the intrapancreatic portion of the bile duct was present causing a dilated intrahepatic biliary tree.

164. Chronic calcific pancreatitis is associated with alcoholism and is a cause of recurrent abdominal pain. An abdominal x-ray in this patient shows pancreatic calcification lying behind the duodenal bulb which is filled with air.

Alcoholic liver disease –
pathological course

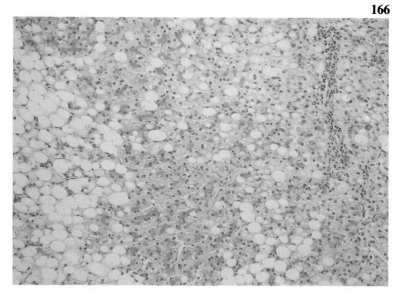

166. Fatty liver develops early in alcoholic liver disease. A biopsy shows most of the liver cells contain large fat droplets. During the processing of this section the fat droplets have dissolved out leaving empty holes. *(H. & E. × 40)*

167

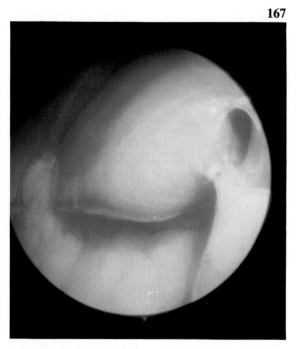

167. Fatty liver. Peritoneoscopy shows an enlarged swollen liver, which is pale due to heavy fatty infiltration.

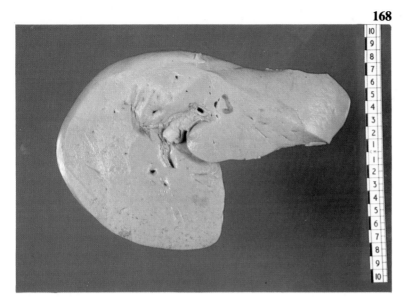

168. Fatty liver. The yellow colour of this liver from an alcoholic is due to massive fatty infiltration.

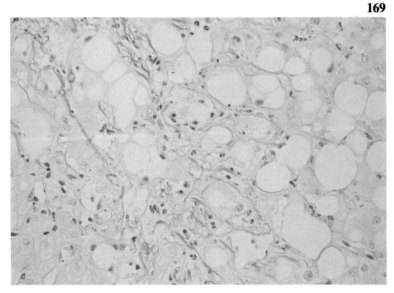

169. Creeping collagenosis. Early in the course of alcoholic liver disease, fine fibrous septa develop around the central veins, following liver cell necrosis. These septa of new collagen extend into the lobule dividing the liver into regular small nodules. The process can eventually lead to a micronodular cirrhosis. This slide shows the early development of creeping collagenosis in a fatty liver. The collagen has been stained pink by van Gieson's method ($\times 100$). This appearance is also known as sclerosing central hyaline necrosis and is an important factor in the development of portal hypertension in alcoholic liver disease.

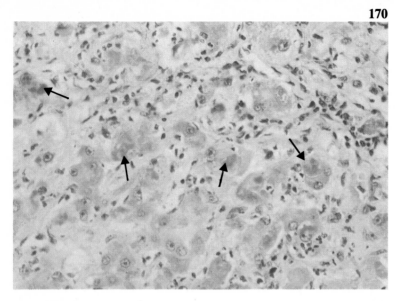

170. Mallory's alcoholic hyaline. In acute alcoholic hepatitis centrizonal liver cell necrosis and acute inflammatory cell infiltration develop, as in any hepatitis. Additionally, the cytoplasm of degenerating liver cells contain irregular clumps of refractile eosinophilic material. This is Mallory's alcoholic hyaline (arrowed). This pink staining material may rarely be found in other chronic liver diseases, but never centrizonally as in alcoholic hepatitis. *(H.&E.×100)*

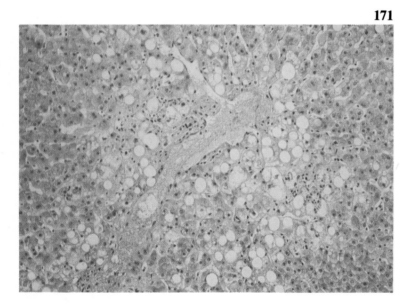

171. Acute alcoholic hepatitis. An acute hepatitis, with liver cell necrosis, inflammatory cell infiltrates, fatty change and alcoholic hyaline is evident around the central vein. There are no signs of cirrhosis. This patient continued to drink. *(H.&E.×40)*

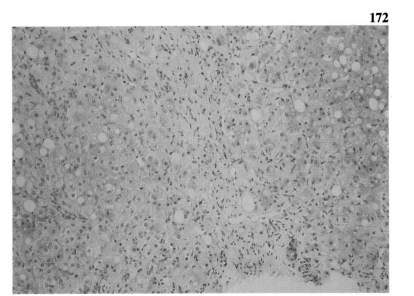

172. Acute alcoholic hepatitis and cirrhosis. Three years later a second biopsy from the patient shown in **171**, demonstrated progression of the liver disease. Now, in addition to alcoholic hepatitis, active fibrous septa are dividing the liver into nodules. An active cirrhosis has developed. The patient then stopped drinking. *(H. & E. ×40)*

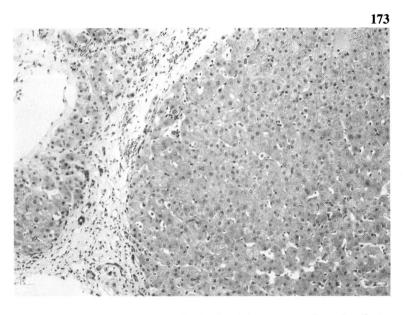

173. Inactive micronodular cirrhosis. Five years after the first biopsy (**171**) a third biopsy in this patient shows an inactive cirrhosis. The inflammation and liver cell necrosis have disappeared and fibrous septa separate small nodules. *(H. & E. ×40)*

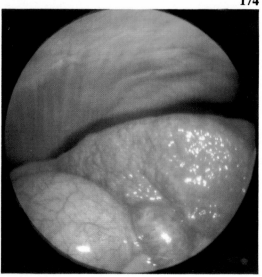

174

174. Peritoneoscopy in a patient with late alcoholic cirrhosis shows a small liver. The surface is finely nodular indicating a micronodular cirrhosis.

Rare causes of cirrhosis

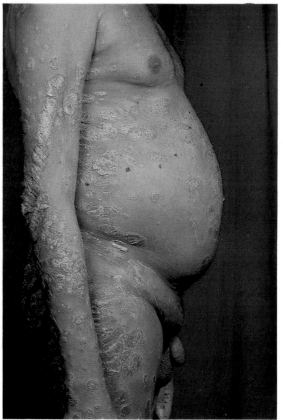

175

175. Methotrexate therapy causes portal zone fibrosis in the liver. During prolonged treatment with methotrexate the portal fibrosis may progress to cirrhosis. This is seen in patients with psoriasis who receive the drug for long periods. The development of cirrhosis is related to both the dose and duration of methotrexate treatment. This psoriatic patient had been on the drug for four years when ascites appeared. Methotrexate therapy had resulted in cirrhosis.

176. Methotrexate. The liver biopsy shows fibrous septa surrounding nodules of liver tissue. Fatty change is present in some hepatocytes but inflammatory cells are conspicuously absent. This is a late stage of methotrexate toxicity, fibrosis alone is more common.

176

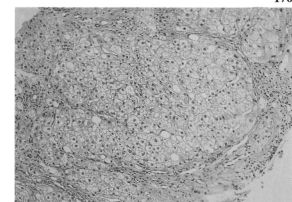

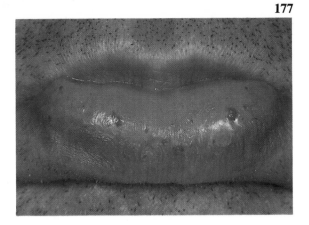

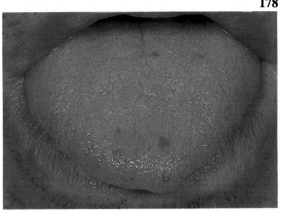

177. Hereditary haemorrhagic telangiectasia. Hepatomegaly is common in this rare disease. Cirrhosis may be due to viral hepatitis contracted from the blood transfusions these patients require. In some cases cirrhosis appears to be associated with the telangiectases. In tnis cirrhotic patient thin walled telangiectases are present on the lips.

178. Hereditary haemorrhagic telangiectasia. Numerous telangiectases are also present on the tongue of the patient in **177**.

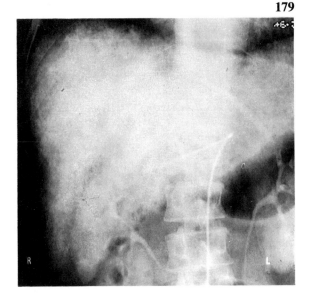

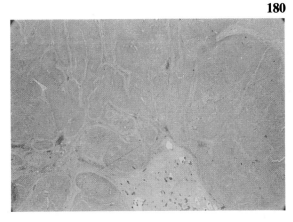

180. Hereditary haemorrhagic telangiectasia. The wedge liver biopsy from the patient in **177** shows an inactive cirrhosis. The fibrous septa surrounding the regenerative nodules contain numerous telangiectases.

179. Hereditary haemorrhagic telangiectasia. The venous phase of a selective coeliac axis arteriogram shows a marked and prolonged venous 'blush' in an enlarged liver. The numerous dense pools of contrast are caused by the telangiectases in the liver.

4. Familial non-haemolytic jaundice

Unconjugated hyperbilirubinaemia

In these patients the serum total bilirubin concentration is above the upper limit of the normal range (greater than 1mg/100ml; 17μmol/l) and most of the bilirubin is unconjugated (non-esterified). However, all other liver function tests are normal. Fasting causes the serum bilirubin level to rise. Gilbert's syndrome is both the commonest and the mildest unconjugated hyperbilirubinaemia. The serum bilirubin level in Gilbert's syndrome rarely exceeds 3mg/100ml (51μmol/l). The prognosis is excellent. Very rarely a severe unconjugated hyperbilirubinaemia is encountered when jaundice is present from birth. This is the Crigler-Najjar syndrome. Most infants affected die in the first year of life from kernicterus. Occasionally these patients develop normally to adult life.

181, 182. Crigler-Najjar syndrome. This man had been deeply jaundiced since birth. The serum total bilirubin concentration varied between 19mg/100ml (323μmol/l) and 21mg/100ml (357μmol/l) and was all unconjugated. Apart from the jaundice, this patient remained in good health.

Phenobarbitone therapy may lower the bilirubin level dramatically in some of these cases. The patient was treated with phenobarbitone and his serum bilirubin concentration fell to 5mg/100ml (85μmol/l).

181

182

Conjugated hyperbilirubinaemia

Chronic intermittent jaundice due to conjugated hyperbilirubinaemia is seen in the Dubin-Johnson and Rotor syndrome. Since the bilirubin is conjugated it appears in the urine. Other liver function tests are normal. The principal distinction between these two syndromes is a darkly pigmented liver in the Dubin-Johnson type. These conditions are benign.

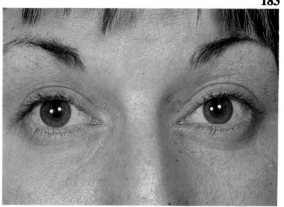

183. Dubin-Johnson syndrome. Clinical jaundice is usually intermittent. It may present during pregnancy or in patients starting the oral contraceptive pill.

184. Dubin-Johnson syndrome. The liver is a greenish-black colour and this striking feature is easily recognised in a liver biopsy. The lower liver biopsy comes from a Dubin-Johnson patient. The upper biopsy is normal.

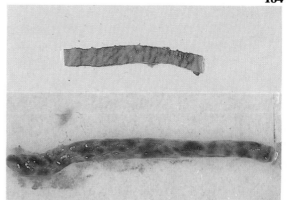

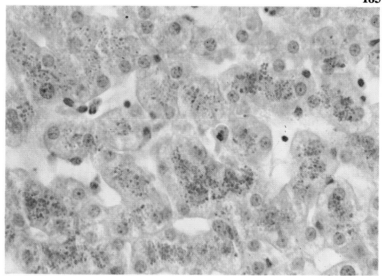

185. Dubin-Johnson syndrome. The dark colour of the liver is due to granules of a brown pigment in the liver cells and Kupffer cells. The pigment is most dense in the centrizonal areas and stains like a lipofuscin. *(H. & E. ×160)*

5. Cholestasis

Cholestasis is defined as the failure of bile flow from the hepatocyte to the duodenum. Previously the term 'obstructive jaundice' was used, but this was inaccurate because in many cholestatic patients no bile duct obstruction can be found. Cholestasis is classified as either *extrahepatic* where there is a mechanical block in the bile ducts or *intrahepatic* where no biliary obstruction is present. Many of the signs of cholestasis are the same irrespective of the cause. Occasionally, associated signs indicate the diagnosis. Examples are a palpable enlarged gall bladder where a cancer of the head of the pancreas obstructs the bile duct, and Sjögrens syndrome in primary biliary cirrhosis. Prolonged cholestasis lasting months or years leads to progressive liver damage and eventually to a biliary cirrhosis with formation of regenerative nodules and fibrosis. The development of a biliary cirrhosis is usually heralded by ascites and signs of hepatocellular failure including portal-systemic encephalopathy.

186. Cholestatic jaundice is a greeny-yellow colour. This patient had a benign traumatic bile duct stricture following a cholecystectomy. *Hepatomegaly* with a firm, non tender edge is usual.

186

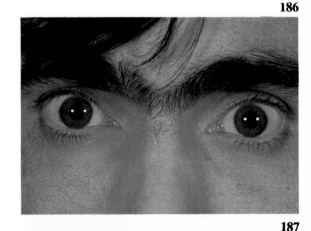

187

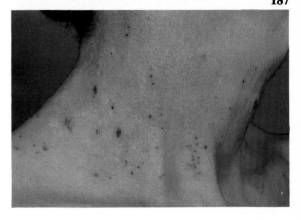

187. Pruritus is another sign of cholestasis. Itching may be intense. In this patient with primary biliary cirrhosis the severe excoriations on her neck resulted from scratching. Pruritus disappears with the onset of liver failure.

188. Thickened skin (lichenification) results from prolonged scratching in patients with chronic cholestasis. Note the xanthomas in the antecubital fossa. They mark the sites of past venepunctures. This patient had primary biliary cirrhosis.

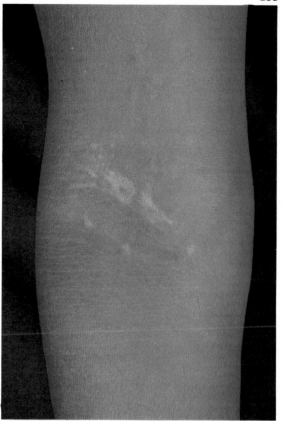

189. Xanthomas. The earliest to develop is xanthelasma, starting in the inner canthus of the eye and spreading laterally. Xanthelasmas are yellow, flat, slightly raised and soft. This patient with primary biliary cirrhosis is also pigmented.

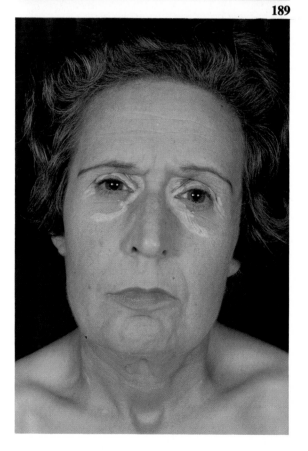

189

190. Xanthomas. Later in the course of a chronic cholestasis tuberous xanthomas may appear. Typically they develop on the extensor surfaces, pressure areas and in scars. The xanthomas on the ear of this patient with primary biliary cirrhosis are related to pressure on the ear lobe when she lies down.

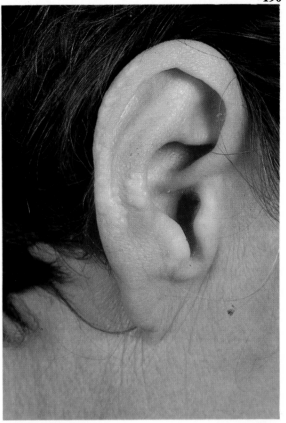

191. Xanthomas. The extensor surfaces of the elbows are a common site for the development of tuberous xanthomas. This patient had primary biliary cirrhosis.

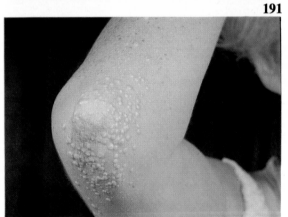

192. Xanthomas. Pressure from a tight-fitting ring caused the circular xanthoma on this finger.

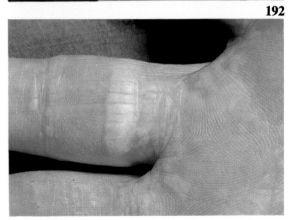

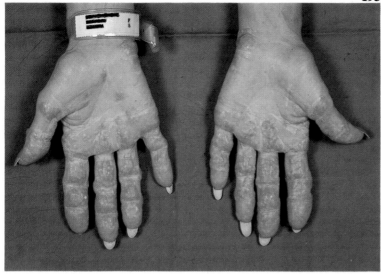

193. Xanthomas commonly develop on the palms. The palmar creases are affected first. Later tuberous xanthomas appear on the fingers. In very severe cases, such as in this patient with primary biliary cirrhosis, finger movements are limited by the xanthomas. In cholestasis tendon sheath xanthomas are rare.

194

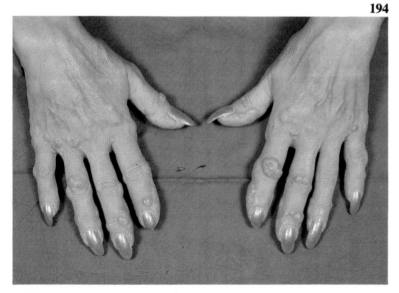

194. Xanthomas. The dorsal surface of the hands of the patient shown in **193** are also covered with large tuberous xanthomas. The fingers are clubbed.

195. Xanthomas. Tuberous xanthomas may develop on the buttocks following constant pressure in this area. This patient had primary biliary cirrhosis.

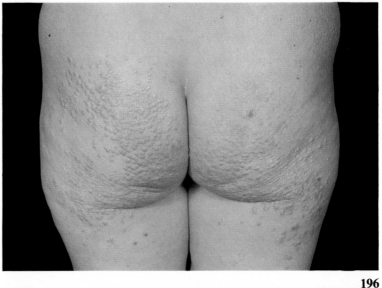

196. Xanthomas. In black patients the bright yellow colour of the xanthoma may be obscured by skin pigmentation. This patient had secondary biliary cirrhosis following a traumatic bile duct stricture. The xanthomas appear as hard raised papules on his buttocks.

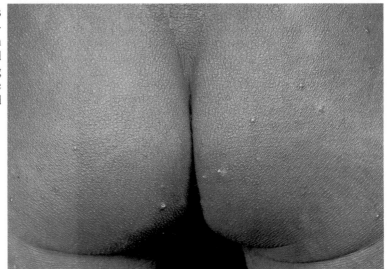

197. Xanthoma. Pressure from shoes caused the raised yellow xanthomatous patches on the first metatarso-phalangeal joint. The patient had primary biliary cirrhosis.

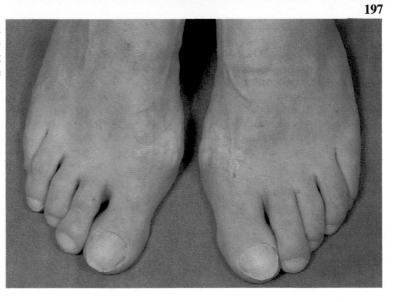

198. Pigmentation of the skin due to increased melanin deposition occurs in patients with prolonged cholestasis. This European patient had primary biliary cirrhosis.

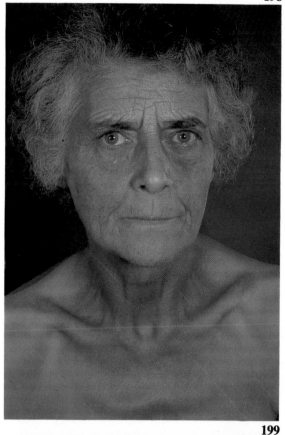

199. Pigmentation of the nails in cholestasis is due to staining with bile pigments. This patient developed nail pigmentation during attacks of benign recurrent intrahepatic cholestasis.

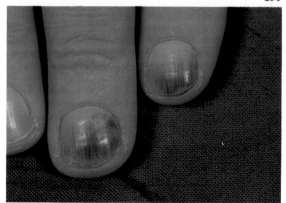

200. Clubbing of the fingers is a common feature of chronic cholestasis. In this patient, with primary biliary cirrhosis, the distal parts of the nails are also pigmented. The proximal parts of the nails are white indicating chronic hepato-cellular failure.

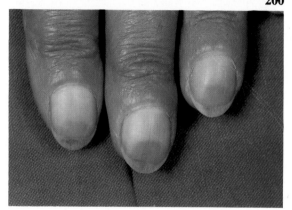

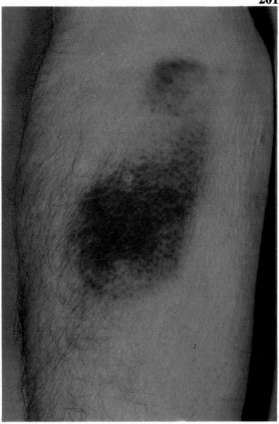

201. Bruising around venepuncture sites is caused by a clotting disorder in cholestasis. The clotting disorder is due to reduced intestinal absorption of vitamin K. This patient had a carcinoma of the bile duct. The prothrombin time was prolonged eight seconds over the control value but returned to normal after vitamin K injections.

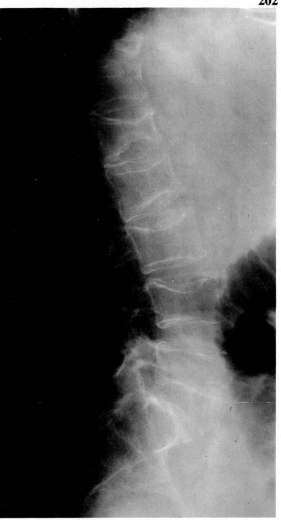

202. Osteomalacia develops in chronic cholestasis due to abnormal calcium and vitamin D metabolism. Demineralisation of the bones has led to crushed and wedge-shaped vertebral bodies in this patient. She had been jaundiced for five years following a benign bile duct stricture. Secondary biliary cirrhosis had developed. Back pain is a prominent complaint. Osteoporosis may also contribute to the bone thinning. Severe osteoporosis develops in cholestatic patients given prednisolone.

203. Osteomalacia. The hands of the patient in 202 show grossly demineralised bones as a result of osteomalacia. Bony erosions are sometimes present, caused by bone xanthomas.

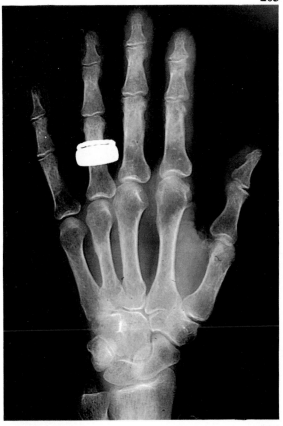

204. Looser's zones are a sign of osteomalacia. This patient with primary biliary cirrhosis suddenly developed pelvic girdle pain without previous trauma. An x-ray of the pelvis shows bands of decalcification in the superior and inferior pubic rami. On either side of the decalcified band are denser shadows of callus. Looser's zones tend to be symmetrical and are also found on the axillary border of the scapula.

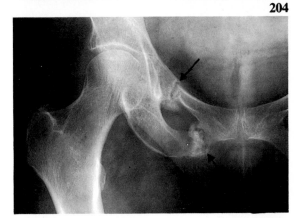

205. Osteomalacia in chronic cholestasis may lead to loosening of the teeth which then fall out. There is resorption of bone around the tooth and the lamina dura disappears. These changes are present in the x-ray (1) from a patient with primary biliary cirrhosis. The adjacent x-ray (2) shows the normal appearance.

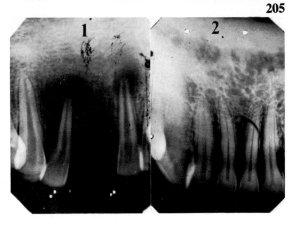

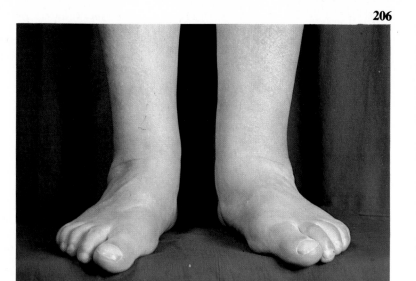 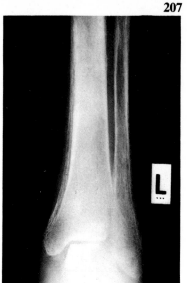

206. Hypertrophic osteoarthropathy may develop in cholestasis causing painful swelling of the wrists and ankles. Hypertrophic osteoarthropathy is responsible for the ankle swelling in this patient with primary biliary cirrhosis.

207. Hypertrophic osteoarthropathy. An x-ray of the ankles of the patient shown in **206** reveals a ring of new subperiostial bone at the lower end of the tibia ('onion skin' appearance).

Investigation of cholestasis

The first objective in the investigation of cholestasis is to determine whether the cause is intrahepatic or extrahepatic. Most cases are due to gallstones (see Chapter 11), cancer of the pancreas and biliary tree or secondary cancer causing extrahepatic cholestasis (see Chapter 10) and viral, drug or alcoholic hepatitis causing intra-hepatic cholestasis (see Chapters 2 and 3).

208. Liver biopsy. Bile pigment (arrow) accumulates in the liver cells, Kupffer cells and the bile canaliculi. The pigment is mainly conjugated bilirubin and is most dense in the centrizonal areas. *(H. & E. ×100)*

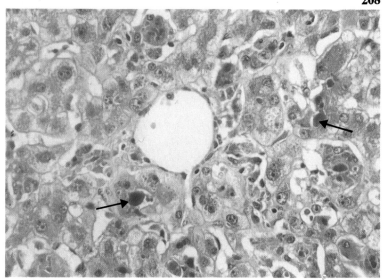

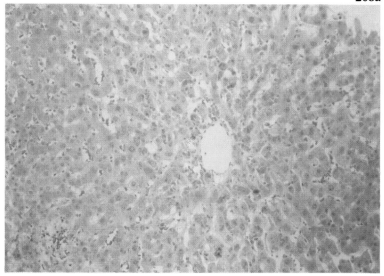

208a. Liver biopsy. The centrizonal distribution of bile pigment in cholestasis is clearly seen in this biopsy. Large amounts of yellow material are deposited around a central vein. *(H. & E. ×40)*

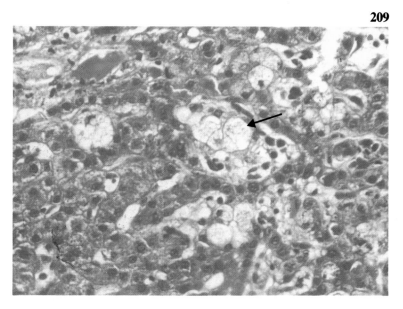

209. Liver biopsy. Some centrizonal liver cells undergo 'feathery' degeneration (arrow) and are surrounded by mononuclear cells. Centrizonal accumulations of bile pigment and 'feathery' degeneration develop in all forms of cholestasis whether intrahepatic or extrahepatic. *(H. & E. ×100)*

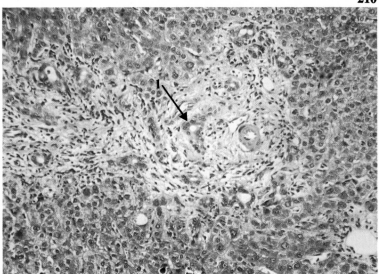

210. Liver biopsy. An extrahepatic cholestasis is usually characterised by marked changes in the portal tracts (1). The bile ducts
proliferate and are tortuous, with a wide lumen. The portal tracts
are enlarged by infiltration with acute inflammatory cells. These are
mainly polymorphonuclears and indicate infection above the
obstruction. Oedema and portal zone fibrosis also develop. In this
patient gallstones were obstructing the common bile duct.
Occasionally, areas of focal liver cell necrosis become bile stained,
forming 'bile lakes'. *(H. & E. ×40)*

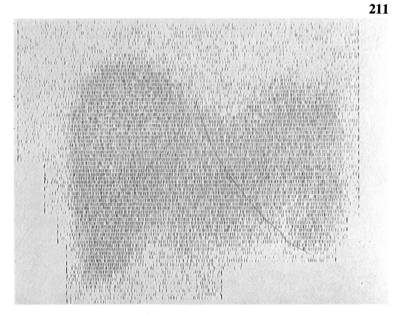

211. Isotope scan in extrahepatic cholestasis may show a filling
defect at the porta hepatis. This is due to dilated intrahepatic bile
ducts which do not take up the ^{99}technetium isotope. This patient
had a cancer of the head of the pancreas obstructing the common
bile duct.

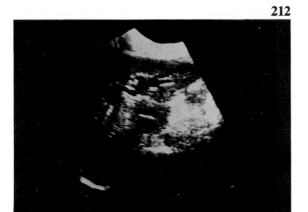

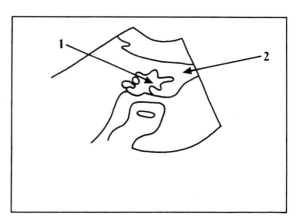

212. Grey scale ultrasonography of the liver in this patient with extrahepatic cholestasis shows a star-shaped filling defect (1) in the liver (2). This is due to dilated intrahepatic bile ducts. A cancer of the head of the pancreas was obstructing the common bile duct. (Scanned 14.5cm above the umbilicus.)

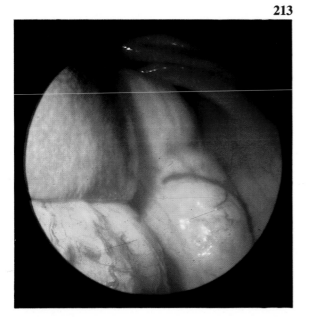

213. Peritoneoscopy in cholestasis shows the liver to be enlarged and green. This patient had a cancer of the head of the pancreas obstructing the bile duct.

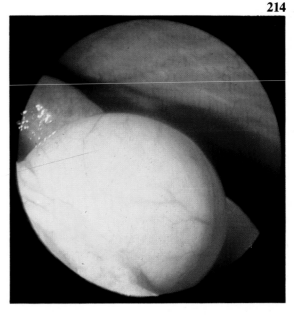

214. Peritoneoscopy. Another view in the patient shown in **213** reveals a tense enlarged gall bladder. This indicates that the bile duct obstruction is below the level of the cystic duct.

215. Percutaneous cholangiography. In this jaundiced patient the needle has entered a grossly dilated intrahepatic biliary system. No contrast flowed down the common bile duct. This obstruction was due to a carcinoma of the bile duct at the porta hepatis.

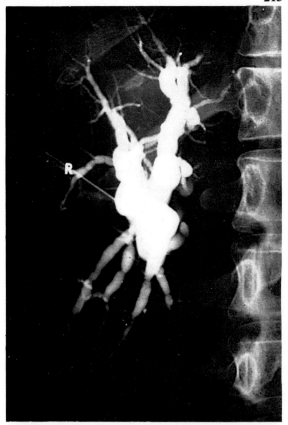

216. Endoscopic retrograde cholangiography is also employed to determine the cause of a cholestasis. In this patient the study revealed a normal common bile duct (1), intrahepatic ducts (2), cystic duct (3) and gall bladder (4). The pancreatic duct (5) was also normal. The cause of the cholestasis was chlorpromazine.

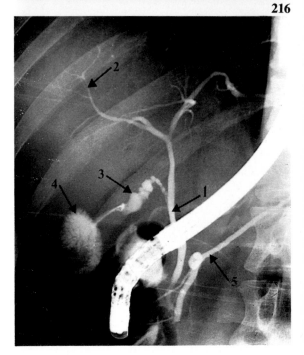

Uncommon causes of cholestasis

1. Ulcerative colitis and Crohn's disease

A variety of hepatobiliary disorders are associated with inflammatory bowel disease. Fatty infiltration in the liver is common.

217

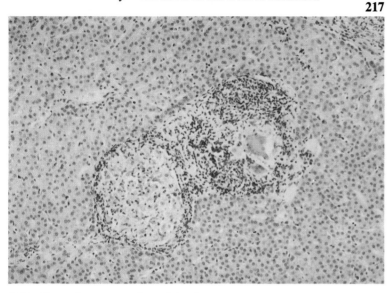

217. Granulomas are found in the liver in both ulcerative colitis and Crohn's disease. These may be well developed with a cuff of lymphocytes enclosing epithelioid cells and giant cells. Caseation does not occur. Alone, they are not usually of clinical significance. *(H. & E. ×40)*

218

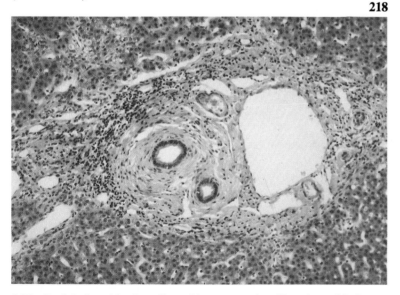

218. Pericholangitis describes this progressive fibrosis and inflammation of the portal tracts. Rings of fibrous tissue enclose the small bile ducts in the portal tracts and there is chronic inflammatory cell infiltration. This is a common finding in ulcerative colitis but is usually asymptomatic. *(H. & E. ×40)*

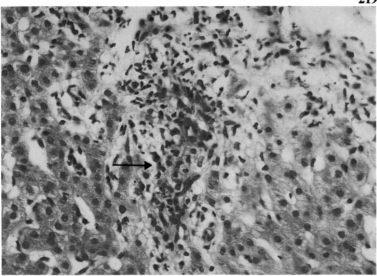

219. Primary sclerosing cholangitis is an uncommon association of both ulcerative colitis and Crohn's disease. Sclerosing cholangitis affects the larger elements of the biliary system so that a liver biopsy only shows the changes of extrahepatic cholestasis. This biopsy, from a patient with primary sclerosing cholangitis, shows acute inflammation of a portal tract with proliferation of bile ductules, indicating large bile duct obstruction. *(H. & E. ×63)*

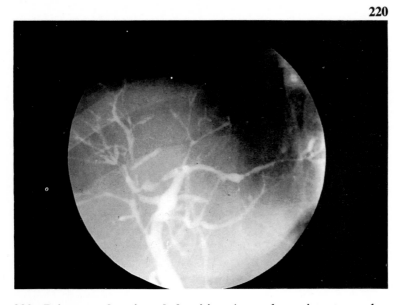

220. Primary sclerosing cholangitis. An endoscopic retrograde cholangiogram in the patient shown in **219** demonstrates the changes of sclerosing cholangitis. The intrahepatic bile ducts are alternately stenosed and dilated resulting in the typical 'beaded' appearance. These patients usually have bouts of fever and jaundice and may develop a constant deep cholestasis. Primary sclerosing cholangitis is also associated with Riedel's struma, mediastinal and retroperitoneal fibrosis, pancreatitis and orbital fibrosis.

221. Carcinoma of the bile ducts is associated with ulcerative colitis and sclerosing cholangitis. This percutaneous cholangiogram from a colitic patient shows the beaded intrahepatic bile ducts of sclerosing cholangitis. The stricture at the porta hepatis (1) is due to a bile duct adenocarcinoma.

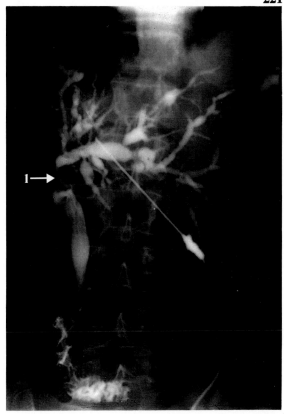

222. Macronodular cirrhosis is an uncommon association with ulcerative colitis. This liver, from a patient with ulcerative colitis, shows the typical large nodules and irregular fibrous septa of a macronodular cirrhosis. Chronic active hepatitis may also be seen.

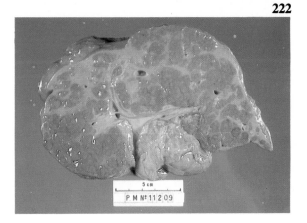

2. Benign recurrent intrahepatic cholestasis

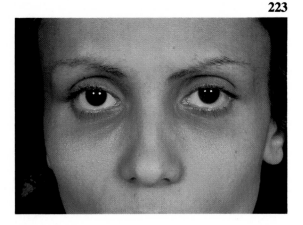

223

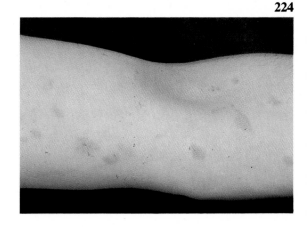

224

223. Benign recurrent intrahepatic cholestasis is rare. The patient suffers repeated attacks of cholestatic jaundice. This was the patient's seventh attack and her serum bilirubin concentration was 21mg/100ml (357µmol/l). The syndrome may be familial. There is no bile duct obstruction. The cholestasis is self-limiting and usually lasts about two months, but this varies.

224. Macular eruption in this man always preceded attacks of benign recurrent intrahepatic cholestasis. A proportion of patients complain of transient rashes on the shoulders and arms associated with the cholestasis.

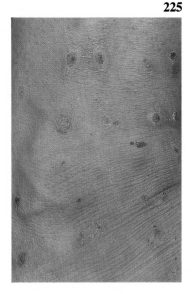

225

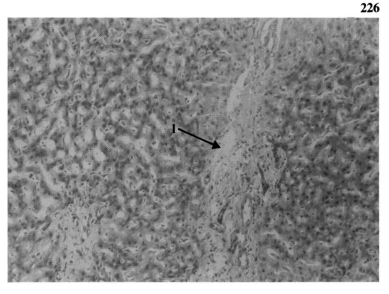

226

225. Pruritus is usually the first sign of a cholestatic attack and appears before the jaundice. The pruritus is often severe and may dominate the patient's illness. The scratch marks on this girl's legs result from severe pruritus.

226. Liver biopsy during the cholestatic attack shows centrizonal cholestasis and moderate mononuclear infiltration of the portal zones. Between attacks the liver is normal apart from mild portal zone fibrosis (1). *(H.&E.×40)*

3. Sickle cell crisis

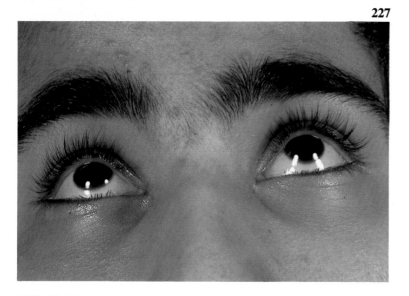

227. Sickle cell crisis may result in a severe intrahepatic cholestasis. Characteristically the serum bilirubin level is enormously increased. In this Arab boy the serum total bilirubin level was 54mg/100ml (918μmol/l); most of the bilirubin was conjugated.

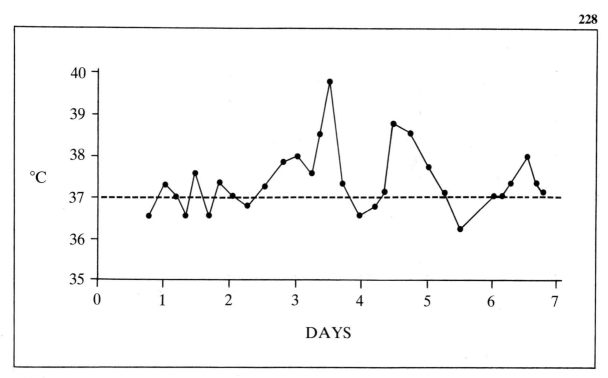

228. Pyrexia. An intermittent pyrexia is commonly present during a sickle cell crisis. Fevers up to 40°C were recorded in the patient shown in **227**. No infective cause could be found for the fever.

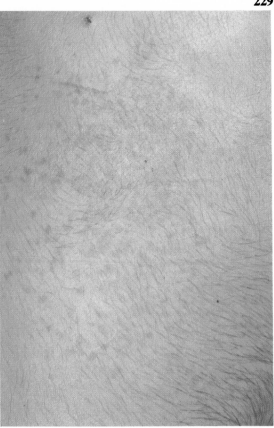

229. Septicaemia. During a sickle cell crisis patients are especially prone to infections. One day before his death this purpuric rash appeared on the abdomen, buttocks and legs of the patient shown in **227**. The purpura was due to gram negative septicaemia. Bone infections also occur.

230

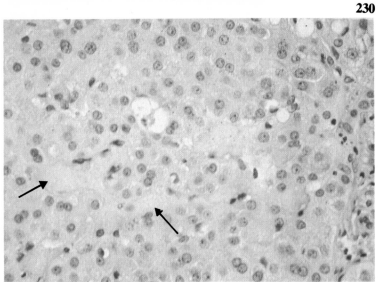

230. Liver biopsy in a sickle cell crisis. The hepatic sinusoids are dilated and full of clumps of sickled red blood cells. *(H. & E. ×100)*

4. Drug-induced cholestasis

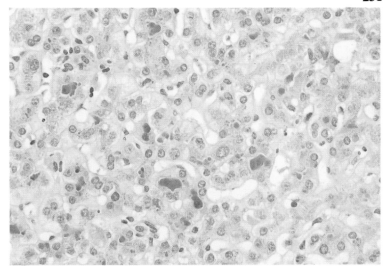

231. Oral contraceptive drugs may rarely cause an intrahepatic cholestasis. The jaundice usually develops by the second cycle. The liver biopsy changes are confined to centrizonal cholestasis. The portal tracts are normal. Recovery follows when the drug is stopped. These patients may also develop cholestasis of late pregnancy. A dose dependent pure cholestasis may also follow ingestion of C17-α substituted testosterones such as methyl testosterone. *(H. & E. ×100)*

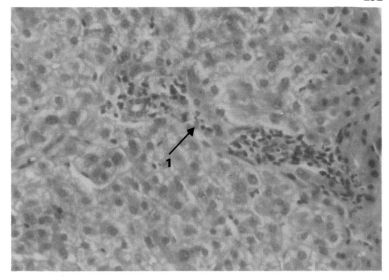

232. Chlorpromazine may cause an intrahepatic cholestasis. The jaundice usually appears by the third week together with signs of a hypersensitivity reaction. The liver biopsy shows centrizonal cholestasis and some 'feathery degeneration' of liver cells. Chlorpromazine causes a portal zone reaction (1) with mononuclear cell and eosinophil infiltration. Complete recovery is usual. A similar hypersensitivity type cholestasis is associated with other phenothiazine derivatives, tolbutamide, anti-thyroid drugs and gold. *(H. & E. ×100)*

5. Haemobilia

233. Haemobilia is a rare cause of an extrahepatic cholestasis. Following a liver biopsy this patient developed blood clots in the bile ducts causing biliary obstruction. An endoscopic retrograde cholangiogram showed filling defects in the common bile duct and gall bladder. Blood was seen to be escaping from the ampulla of vater.

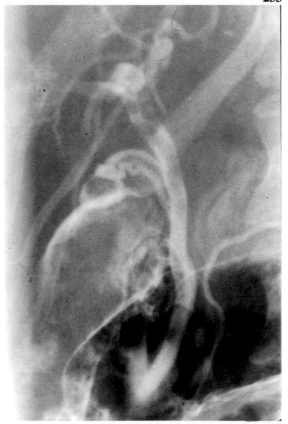

6. Primary biliary cirrhosis
(also called chronic non-suppurative destructive cholangitis and 'Hanot's cirrhosis')

Primary biliary cirrhosis mainly affects women, usually between the ages of 40 and 59 years. The onset is insidious and typically pruritus is the first symptom. Months or years later cholestatic jaundice appears. Pigmentation of the skin and xanthomas are common. A serum mitochondrial antibody is found in 83–98% of patients. Some collagen diseases are associated with primary biliary cirrhosis including Sjögren's syndrome, Raynaud's phenomenon, rheumatoid arthritis, dermatomyositis and scleroderma. Autoimmune thyroiditis and renal tubular acidosis also occur.

234. Primary biliary cirrhosis. The patient is well nourished, mildly jaundiced and pigmented. Hepato-splenomegaly is usual.

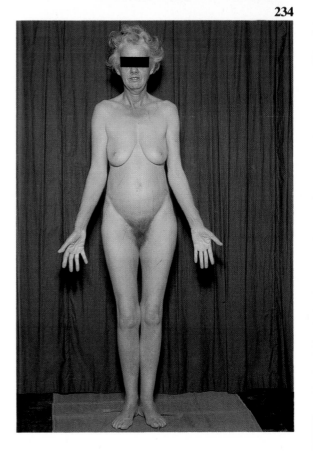

235. Pruritus is often severe in primary biliary cirrhosis. This patient has scratch marks on her back, which is also pigmented. Note the 'butterfly sign' (arrows), an area which has escaped pigmentation on her scapulae. There are no scratch marks in this area. Terminally the pruritus usually disappears.

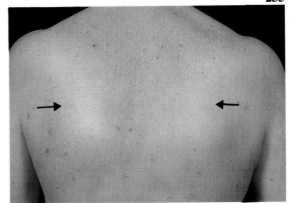

236. Vitiligo. Patchy depigmentation and hyperpigmentation occasionally develop in primary biliary cirrhosis.

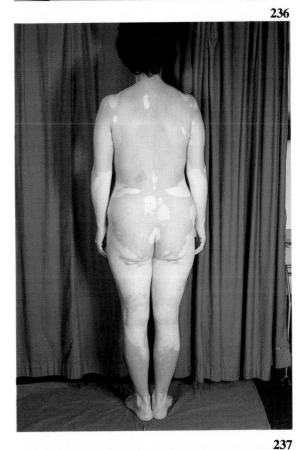

237. Arthritis. The late changes of rheumatoid arthritis have developed in this patient with primary biliary cirrhosis. There is ulnar deviation of the hand, subluxation of the metacarpophalangeal joints and wasting of the small muscles of the hand.

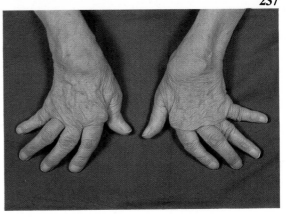

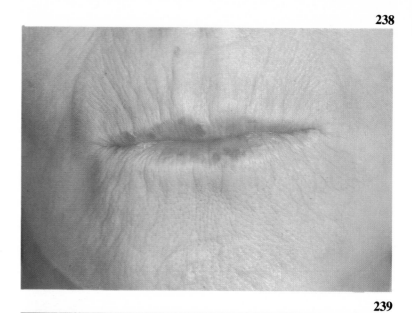

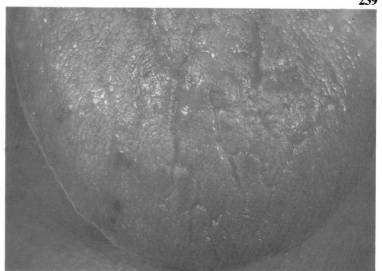

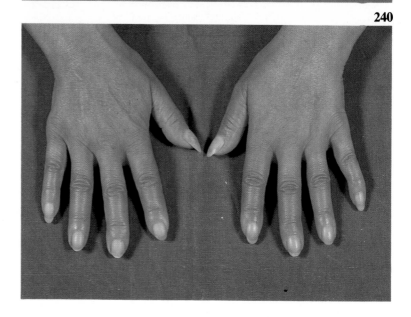

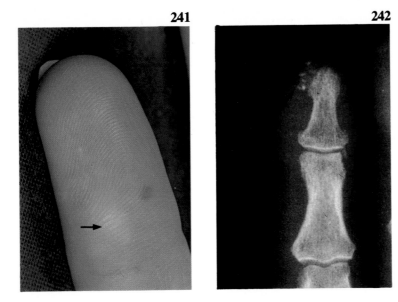

238–242. CRST syndrome. The syndrome comprises calcinosis, Raynaud's phenomenon, sclerodactyly and telangiectasia. Telangiectases are present on the lips (**238**) and tongue (**239**) of this patient with primary biliary cirrhosis. Other sites include the palate, forehead and hands.

Sclerodactyly is the cause of the thickened shiny skin on the patient's fingers. In the later stages the skin atrophies and the fingers become spindle-shaped.

Calcinosis, which are small white patches of subcutaneous calcification (**241**), are present on the patient's finger (arrowed). A telangiectasis can also be seen. An x-ray (**242**) of the finger shows the calcinosis as spotty subcutaneous calcification adjacent to the distal phalanx.

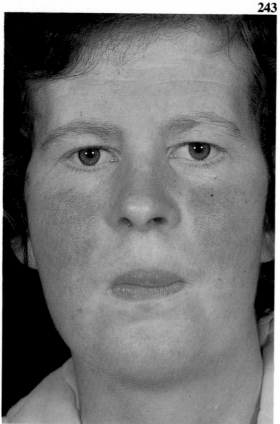

243. Dermatomyositis may be associated with primary biliary cirrhosis. The patient developed the typical lilac coloured (heliotrope) rash on her cheeks and over the bridge of her nose. Periorbital oedema is usually marked. Her main complaint was profound muscle weakness due to a proximal myopathy.

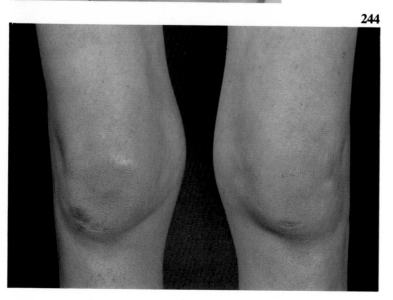

244. Dermatomyositis. The itchy dermatitis was also present on the knees of the patient shown in **243**. Note the wasting of quadriceps femoris due to a proximal myopathy.

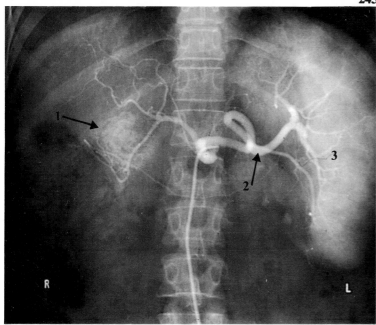

245. Gastric haemangioma is a rare cause of blood loss and anaemia in primary biliary cirrhosis. More commonly gastro-intestinal haemorrhage is due to oesophageal varices or a duodenal ulcer. This patient had an extensive sub-mucosal haemangioma in the antrum of the stomach. The haemangioma was seen as a vascular blush (1) in a coeliac axis arteriogram. The splenic artery (2) has filled an enlarged spleen (3). Splenomegaly is usual in primary biliary cirrhosis.

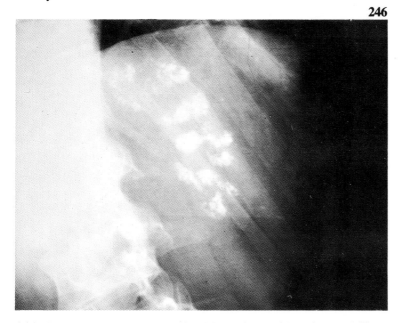

246. Renal tubular acidosis in this patient with primary biliary cirrhosis has resulted in extensive spotty calcification in the renal medulla. Such florid cases are rare, usually renal tubular acidosis is mild and clinically insignificant in primary biliary cirrhosis.

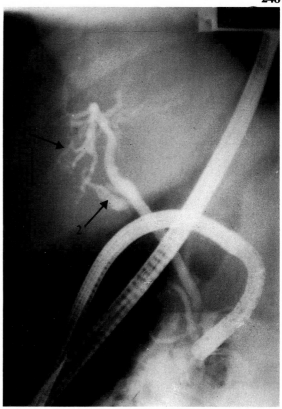

247. Biliary system. Primary biliary cirrhosis only affects the very small bile ducts in the liver. The larger elements of the biliary system are normal unless cirrhosis has developed when their course is distorted by nodule formation. This endoscopic retrograde cholangiogram from a patient with primary biliary cirrhosis shows normal smoothly tapering intrahepatic bile ducts (1). The common bile duct (2), gall bladder (3) and pancreatic duct (4) are all normal. In this patient cirrhosis had not developed.

248. Biliary system. The intrahepatic bile ducts (1) are pruned and their course is tortuous in this patient with primary biliary cirrhosis. The intrahepatic bile ducts have been distorted by cirrhotic nodules. Note the shrunken gall bladder (2) which contains small stones. Patients with primary biliary cirrhosis often develop gallstones.

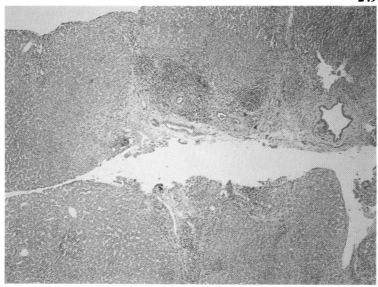

249. Primary biliary cirrhosis. The liver biopsy shows heavy infiltration of the portal tracts with lymphocytes, histiocytes and epithelioid cells. Lymphoid follicles with germinal centres and granulomas may form in the portal tracts in relation to damaged bile ducts. Fibrosis begins in the portal tracts and fibrous septa later spread into and around the lobules. Primary biliary cirrhosis involves the septal and larger interlobular bile ducts so that if these are not included in the biopsy, the characteristic changes may be missed. *(H. & E. ×10)*

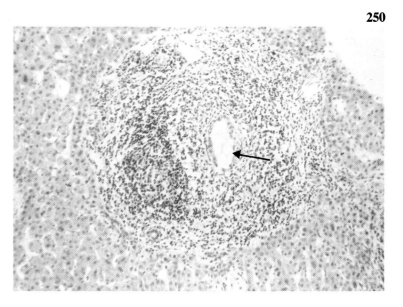

250. Primary biliary cirrhosis. At higher magnification the pathognomonic sign of primary biliary cirrhosis is seen. An enlarged portal tract is infiltrated with chronic inflammatory cells and contains a granuloma adjacent to a damaged bile duct (arrowed). *(H. & E. ×64)*

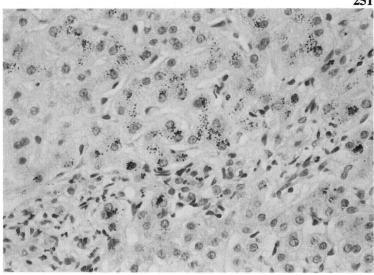

251. Primary biliary cirrhosis. Copper accumulates in the liver cells in any prolonged cholestasis. This is due to impaired biliary excretion of copper. The rhodanine stain shows a heavy load of copper binding protein as red granular deposits in the liver cells of a patient with primary biliary cirrhosis. *(×100)*

252

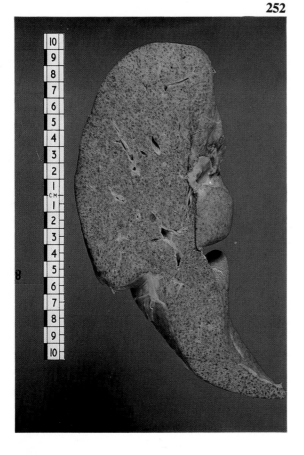

252. Primary biliary cirrhosis. At autopsy the liver is enlarged, green and coarsely nodular.

7. Secondary biliary cirrhosis

Prolonged extrahepatic biliary obstruction may result in secondary biliary cirrhosis. This is most commonly due to a benign bile duct stricture or to gallstones. Malignant strictures of the bile duct, such as cancer of the head of the pancreas, rarely lead to secondary biliary cirrhosis. The patient usually dies from the cancer before biliary cirrhosis has had time to develop.

253, 254. Benign biliary stricture usually follows a cholecystectomy. The jaundice is cholestatic and of variable intensity and is often accompanied by fevers and pain due to cholangitis. This patient has a biliary stricture following a cholecystectomy. The serum bilirubin level was 18mg/100ml (306µmol/l).

Recurrent cholangitis caused temperatures up to 39.5°C in this patient (Charcot's intermittent biliary fever). During the fevers the white blood cell count rose to 24,000mm³ and were predominantly polymorphonuclear leucocytes. *E. coli* were cultured from the blood.

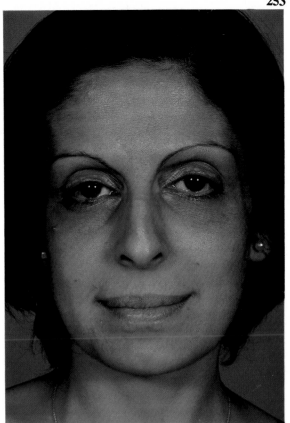

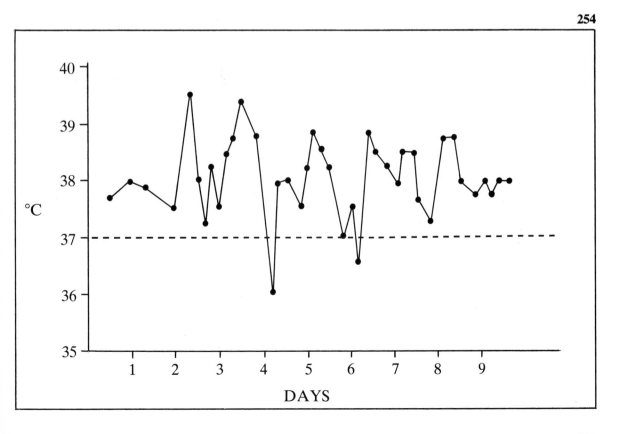

254

255. Benign biliary stricture. A percutaneous cholangiogram from the patient in **253** shows a dilated intrahepatic biliary tree above a tight stricture of the common bile duct. A collection of contrast has accumulated in the gall bladder bed.

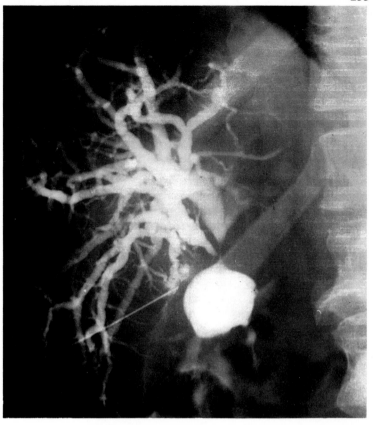

256. Benign biliary stricture. The abdominal walls of these patients are typically marked by many scars which have followed repeated surgical attempts to repair the stricture. This patient had had a biliary stricture for 11 years.

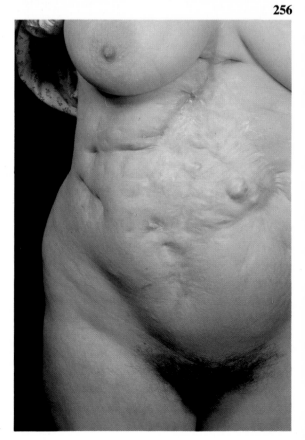

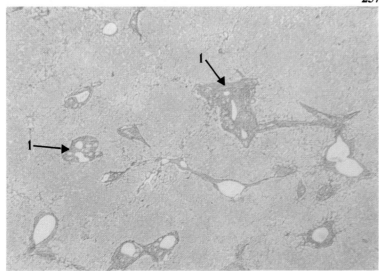

257. Benign biliary stricture in the patient shown in **256** has led to secondary biliary fibrosis. The reticulin stain shows portal fibrosis (1) and septa extending to link portal tracts and central veins. (×10)

258

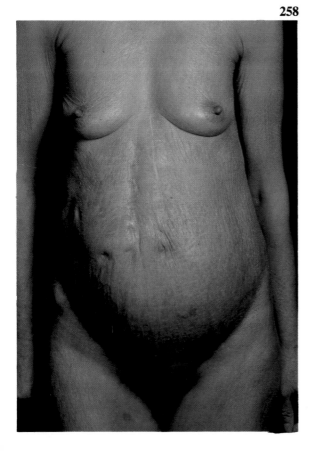

258. Decompensated biliary cirrhosis may be the end result of a benign bile duct stricture. Chronic cholestasis has led to pigmentation in this patient and the ascites indicates a decompensated cirrhosis. Hepato-splenomegaly was present. She suffered repeated attacks of cholangitis

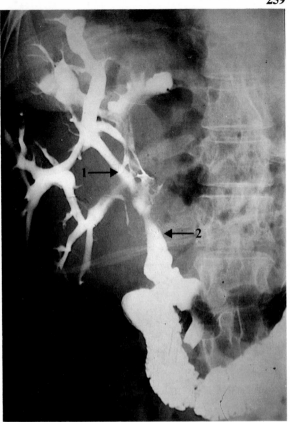

259. Secondary sclerosing cholangitis has developed in the patient shown in **258** as a result of repeated biliary tract infections. The percutaneous cholangiogram shows saccular dilatations and stenoses of the intrahepatic bile ducts indicating secondary sclerosing cholangitis. The anastomosis between the bile duct (1) and jejenum (2) is patent.

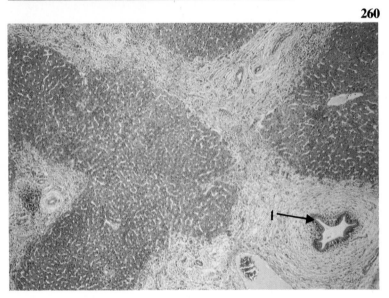

260. Secondary biliary cirrhosis was fully developed in the patient shown in **258**. Extensive portal fibrosis was present. This is especially obvious around a large bile duct (1). Fibrous septa have spread out to link portal tracts, isolating nodules of liver cells. Note the clear margins of the nodules; there is no piecemeal necrosis. *(H. & E. ×24)*

8. Cholestatic syndromes in childhood

Biliary atresia is agenesis or malformation of the biliary tract.

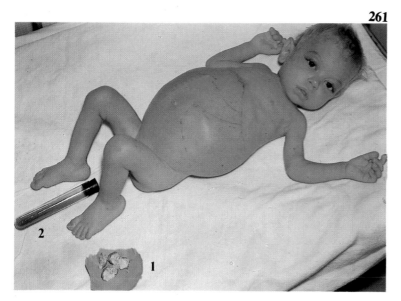

261. **Biliary atresia.** This child is deeply jaundiced and pigmented. Bile is not secreted into the intestine so the stools (1) are pale and the urine (2) dark. Note the grossly enlarged liver which is indenting the abdominal wall. Ascites and portal hypertension are late features. These children usually die by six months.

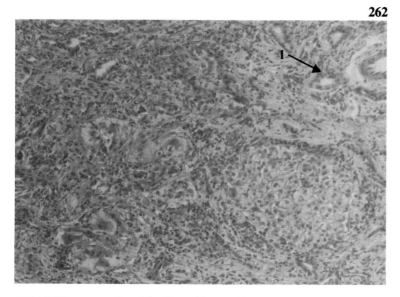

262. **Biliary atresia.** The liver biopsy shows a severe cholestasis, which is mainly centrizonal. Bile plugs are present in the biliary canaliculi. In the portal tracts (1) there is bile ductular proliferation. Giant cells are common, making the distinction from neonatal hepatitis difficult. At laparotomy the bile ducts may be absent or replaced by fibrous strands. *(H. & E. ×70)*

Intrahepatic cholestasis describes children with destruction or absence of the intrahepatic bile ducts.

263, 264. Intrahepatic cholestasis. The infants are usually jaundiced in the neonatal period, but presentation may be delayed until later in childhood. This infant was jaundiced as a neonate. When one year old he presented with xanthomas and pruritus. A xanthelasma is present on the upper eyelid, but the child is not jaundiced. Xanthomas are present on the hands (**264**).

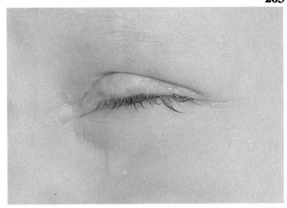

263

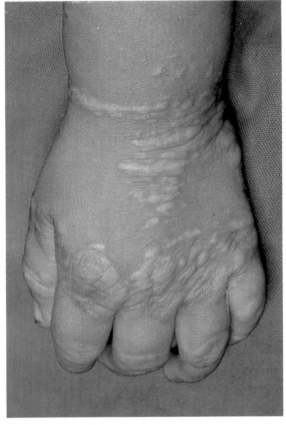

264

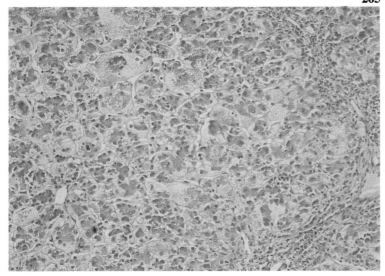

265. Intrahepatic cholestasis. The liver biopsy shows a prominent giant cell reaction. In the portal tracts bile ductules are reduced or absent. *(H. & E. ×40)*

266 **267**

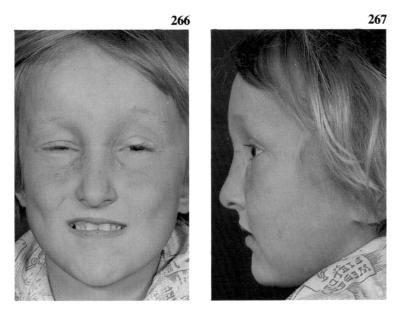

266, 267. Intrahepatic cholestasis. Aged 9, the child shown in **263** was still well. This syndrome usually pursues a more benign course than extrahepatic biliary atresia. A side view shows the flattened facies characteristic of this syndrome.

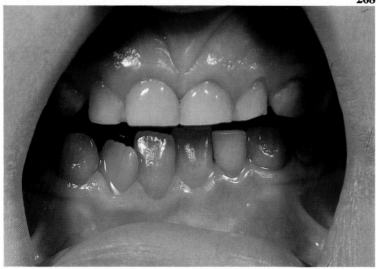

268. Pigmentation of the teeth may develop in children with intra-hepatic cholestasis. This is due to staining of the growing teeth with bile pigments.

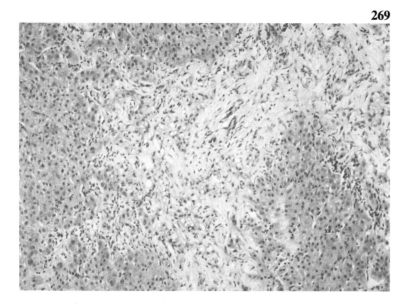

269. Secondary biliary cirrhosis developed in the child shown in **266**. However, progression to cirrhosis is not inevitable in these patients. Thick fibrous septa separate well demarcated nodules in this biopsy. No bile ducts can be seen. The cirrhosis resulted in portal hyper-tension and bleeding from oesophageal varices. *(H. & E. ×40)*

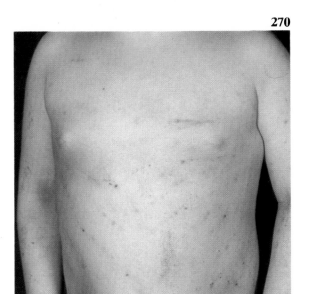

270. Pruritus may be intense in children with intrahepatic cholestasis. This six-year-old girl was not clinically jaundiced but pruritus led to these extensive scratch marks.

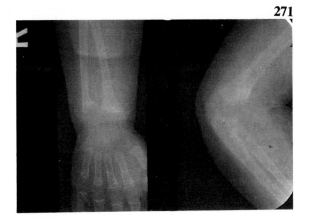

271. Biliary rickets may complicate intrahepatic cholestasis of childhood. The general density of the bones is reduced. The metaphyses are widened and 'cupped' and the depth of the epiphyseal cartilage is increased.

272. Biliary rickets. The widening of the epiphyses and cupping of the metaphyses due to biliary rickets are seen in the femur from a case of intrahepatic cholestasis. Note the green staining of the bone.

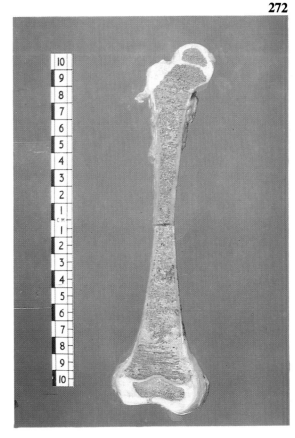

6. Vascular diseases

Portal hypertension

Venous blood from the gastrointestinal tract flows back to the liver through the portal venous system. The inferior mesenteric vein usually enters the splenic vein. The union of the splenic vein and the superior mesenteric vein forms the portal vein. On entering the liver, at the porta hepatis, the portal vein divides into right and left branches to the major lobes of the liver. The umbilical vein joins the left branch of the portal vein.

273. Normal splenic venogram obtained by percutaneous injection of contrast material into the spleen. All the contrast in the spleen (1) rapidly flows through the splenic vein (2) and portal vein (3) into the liver. Note the smoothly tapering intrahepatic portal veins (4) extending to the periphery of the liver. This normal liver has a large Riedel's lobe (arrowed).

Obstruction to the portal venous system results in portal hypertension. The obstruction may be *intrahepatic* (most commonly due to cirrhosis) or *extrahepatic* due to blockage of the portal vein. In response to portal hypertension an extensive collateral circulation develops, draining portal venous blood into the systemic veins. The collateral circulation at the cardia of the stomach leads to oesophageal and gastric varices, and at the anus haemorrhoids may develop. Other sites include the umbilical veins in the falciform ligament, veins from the liver to the diaphragm, veins in the lieno-renal ligament and collaterals to the left renal vein. Patients with portal hypertension usually present with gastro-intestinal haemorrhage from oesophageal varices. In cirrhotic patients bleeding may cause decompensation of the liver disease and ascites, jaundice and portal-systemic encephalopathy develop. With a very large collateral circulation the portal pressure may fall and the liver shrinks.

273

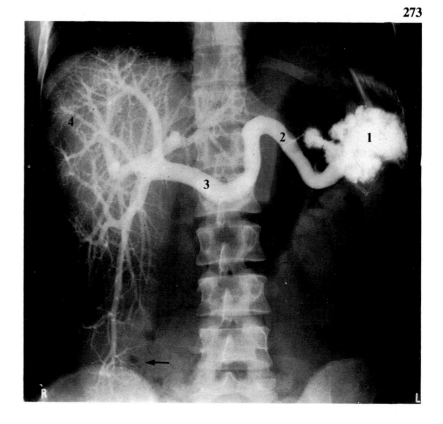

Intrahepatic portal hypertension

274. Splenomegaly is an important sign of portal hypertension. The spleen progressively enlarges as the portal pressure rises. This patient had cirrhosis following chronic active hepatitis and presented with a haematemesis from ruptured oesophageal varices. Regenerating nodules in the liver obstruct the portal venous blood flow. Note the scanty body hair.

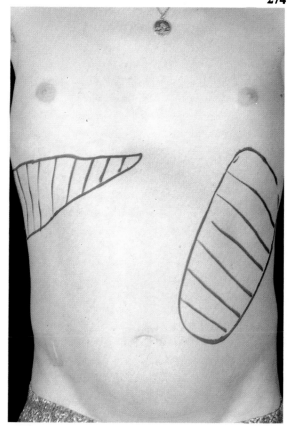

275. Abdominal wall veins in this alcoholic cirrhotic were due to a collateral circulation between the left branch of the portal vein via the umbilical vein and the systemic veins on the anterior abdominal wall. The direction of blood flow is away from the umbilicus. The blue colour of the umbilicus is due to a large vein. Stigmata of chronic liver disease, gynaecomastia and reduced body hair, are also present.

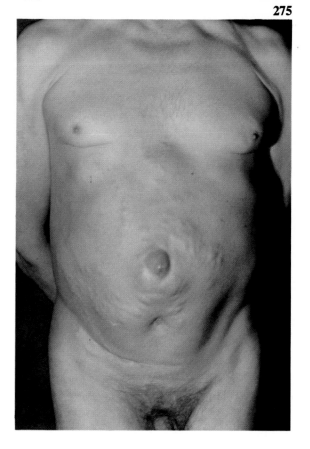

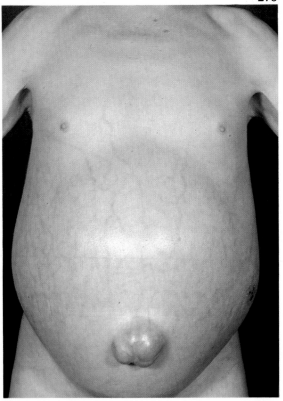 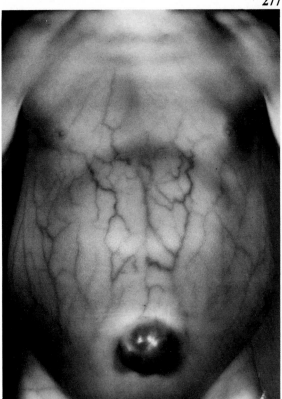

276, 277. Abdominal wall veins. The veins on the abdomen of this alcoholic cirrhotic are portal systemic shunts. Ascites is present and the umbilicus has herniated. Vascular spiders are seen in the necklace area.

An infra-red photograph (**277**) of the patient shows much more clearly the extent of the portal-systemic collaterals on the abdominal wall.

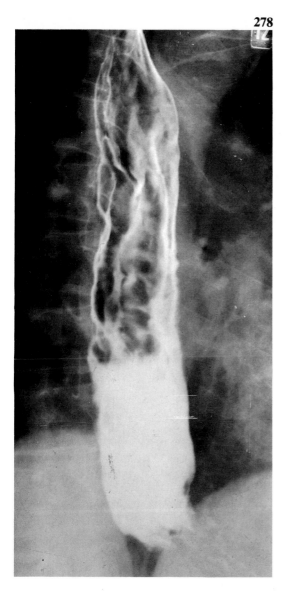

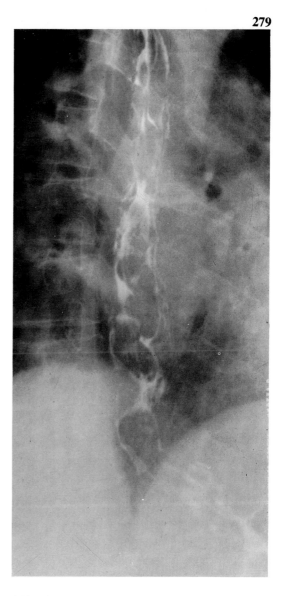

278. Oesophageal varices. Submucosal varices in the oesophagus can be demonstrated radiologically by a barium swallow examination. The x-ray shows a dilated oesophagus which contains thick worm-like filling defects representing the varices.

279. Oesophageal varices are best demonstrated with very little barium in the oesophagus. This x-ray comes from the barium swallow shown in **278**. The worm-like filling defects caused by oesophageal varices are now seen extending the whole length of the oesophagus.

280. Oesophageal varices. Fibreoptic endoscopy is also employed to detect oesophageal varices. This endoscopic picture of the lower end of the oesophagus shows large tortuous dark blue sub-mucosal varices (arrow). This technique will also reveal whether the oesophageal varices are bleeding.

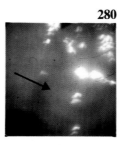

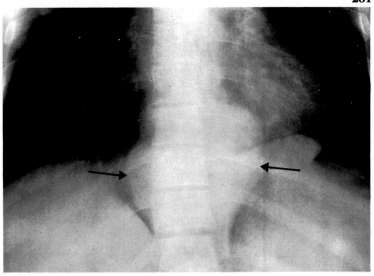

281. Oesophageal varices. Rarely very large varices can be seen in a well penetrated x-ray of the chest. The mass in the lower part of the mediastinum in this patient is due to oesophageal varices.

282

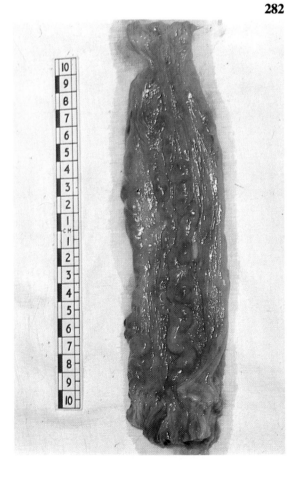

282. Oesophageal varices usually collapse at autopsy so that grossly distended varices are rarely seen. This oesophagus has been laid open and the sinuous dark purple varices can be seen lying under the oesophageal mucosa.

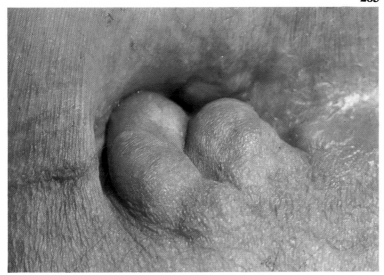

283. Haemorrhoidal varices have developed in this cirrhotic patient. They represent the collateral circulation between the superior haemorrhoidal vein of the portal system and the middle and inferior haemorrhoidal veins of the systemic venous system.

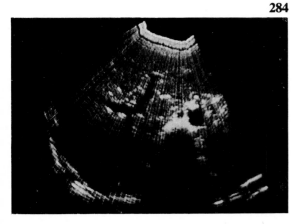
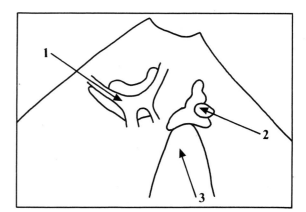

284. Grey scale ultrasonography. Intrahepatic portal hypertension causes dilation of the portal vein (1) which can be shown by ultrasonography. The aorta (2) and a vertebral body (3) are also shown. The portal vein cannot be identified in cases of portal vein thrombosis. Ultrasonography is a useful non-invasive technique to distinguish between intrahepatic and extrahepatic portal hypertension.

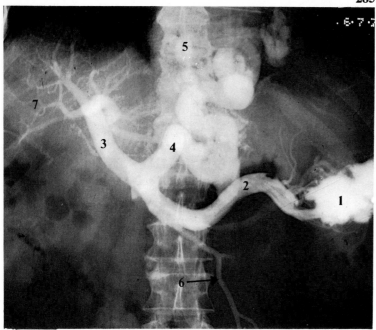

285. Splenic venogram from a patient with portal hypertension due to alcoholic cirrhosis. Injection of contrast into the enlarged spleen (1) has filled the splenic vein (2) and portal vein (3). A large proportion of the contrast is diverted via a dilated and tortuous left gastric vein (4) into a leash of gastric and oesophageal varices (5). There is retrograde flow of contrast down the inferior mesenteric vein (6). The intrahepatic portal veins (7) are pruned, indicating cirrhosis ('tree in winter' appearance).

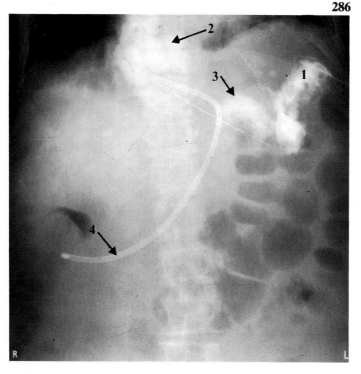

286. Splenic venogram in a cirrhotic patient with actively bleeding varices. Nine seconds after splenic injection (1) contrast is still present in the oesophageal varices (2) and is extravasating into the stomach (3) due to variceal haemorrhage. A naso-gastric tube (4) is in the stomach.

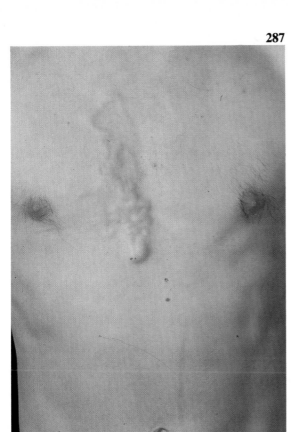

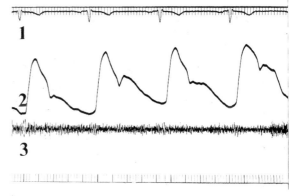

287

288

287, 288. Venous hum was heard over these portal-systemic collaterals at the lower end of the sternum. The patient had cirrhosis following chronic active hepatitis. The spleen was enlarged. The hum was due to blood flow through a large umbilical vein in the falciform ligament supplied by the left branch of the portal vein.

A phonocardiogram (**288**) recorded over the site of the venous hum shows a continuous low pitched noise (3) unrelated to the electrocardiogram (1) or the carotid pulse (2).

289

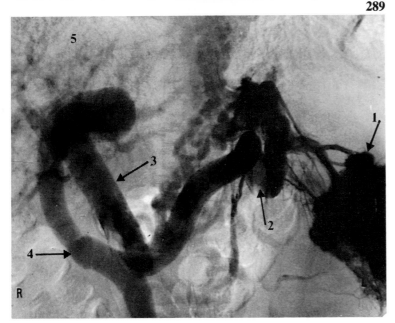

289. Splenic venogram from the patient shown in **287**. Splenic injection (1) has filled the splenic vein (2) and portal vein (3). Most of the contrast flowed down the left branch of the portal vein into a very large umbilical vein (4) and little entered the liver (5). The clarity of this x-ray has been achieved by the use of a 'subtraction' technique.

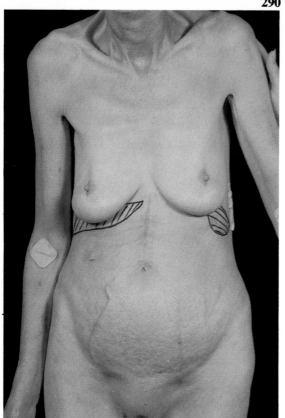

290, 291. Chronic dementia due to portal-systemic encephalopathy is a rare complication of a large collateral circulation in cirrhotic patients. This patient presented with dementia. She had a small inactive cirrhotic liver. The portal vein pressure was normal due to the large portal systemic shunt, hence the spleen was not enlarged. Note the veins on the abdominal wall which are portal systemic collaterals.

The splenic venogram (**291**) shows a very large shunt from the left branch of the portal vein (1) down the umbilical vein (2). Later films showed the umbilical vein draining via the iliac veins into the inferior vena cava. Only a few oesophageal varices (3) have filled, reflecting the decompression of the portal venous system down the umbilical vein.

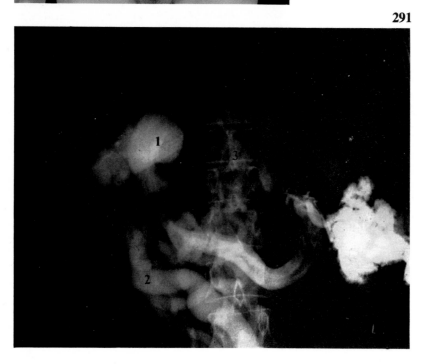

291

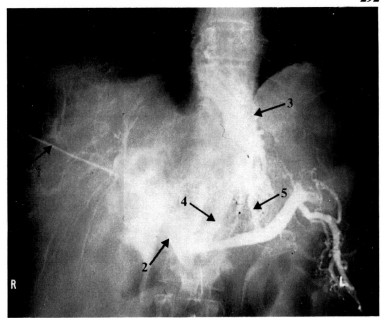

292. Percutaneous transhepatic venography may be used to study the portal venous system. A fine cannula is passed through the liver until the portal vein is entered. By advancing the catheter individual collaterals may be cannulated. In this patient with primary biliary cirrhosis the catheter (1) has passed through the liver into the portal vein (2). A large leash of oesophageal and gastric varices (3) are supplied by the left gastric vein (4) and short gastric veins (5).

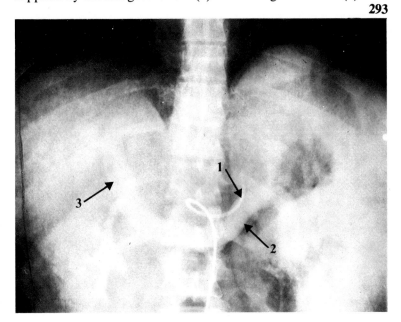

293. Coeliac axis arteriography. The portal venous system may be seen in the venous phase of a coeliac axis arteriogram. However, this technique does not usually opacify the portal venous system as well as splenic venography. In this cirrhotic patient, the catheter has been placed in the splenic artery (1). The venous phase of this study shows the splenic vein (2) and portal vein (3).

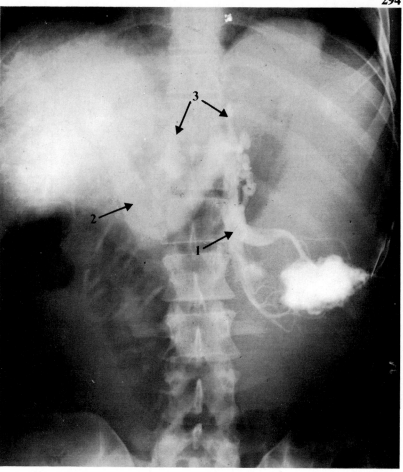

294, 295. Surgery for portal hypertension. A variety of surgical shunts between the portal venous system and the systemic veins are employed to reduce portal hypertension. Intrahepatic portal hypertension due to schistosomiasis resulted in several major haematemeses from oesophageal varices in this patient. The splenic venogram showed a patent splenic vein (1) and portal vein (2) feeding shunts (3) to oesophageal varices.

A shunt between the superior mesenteric vein and the inferior vena cava (a meso-caval shunt) was performed in this patient. A second splenic venogram (**295**) showed much of the blood diverted down the superior mesenteric vein (4) which is draining into the inferior vena cava (5). Note that the portal blood supply to the liver (6) is reduced and that the oesophageal varices no longer fill.

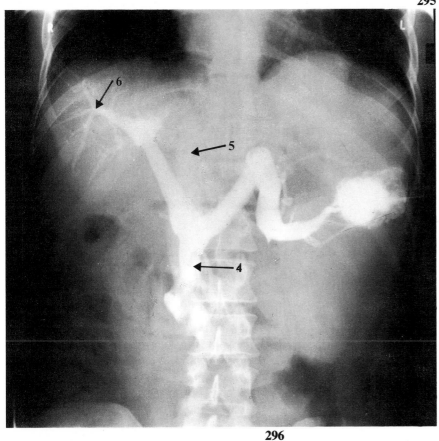

296

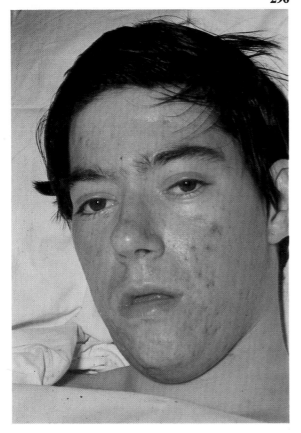

296. Portal-systemic encephalopathy is an important complication of porta-caval shunts. This cirrhotic patient underwent a porta-caval shunt for recurrent variceal haemorrhage. Subsequently he became drowsy with a fetor and a coarse flapping tremor.

Rare causes of intrahepatic portal hypertension

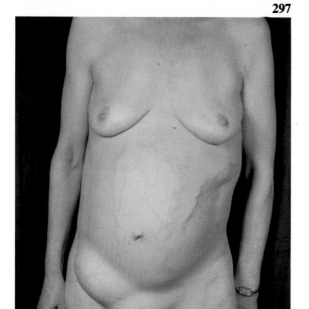

297. Partial nodular transformation is a rare cause of portal hypertension. The hilum of the liver is replaced by nodules. The remainder of the liver is normal. The hilar nodules compress the portal vein resulting in portal hypertension. This patient had partial nodular transformation of the liver. Note the portal systemic shunts on the abdominal wall and the hernias.

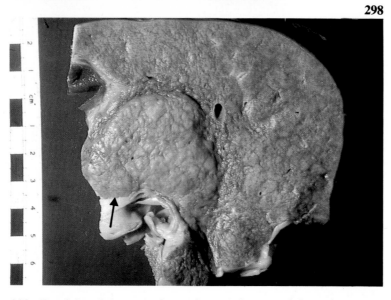

298. Partial nodular transformation. A large nodule at the porta hepatis obstructed the portal vein and caused portal hypertension in this patient. The remainder of the liver was normal.

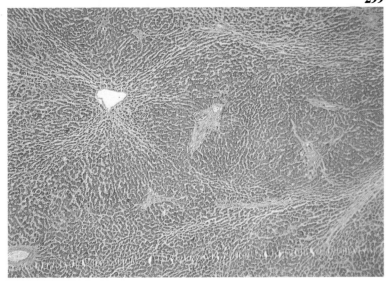

299. Partial nodular transformation. A biopsy of the nodule in **298** showed the liver dissected by slender fibrous septa. The hepatic architecture in the nodule is not grossly disorganised as in cirrhosis. *(H. & E. ×10)*

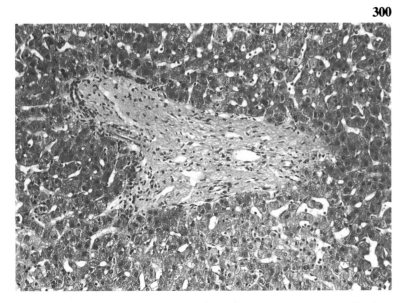

300. Hepatoportal sclerosis or sclerosis of the portal veins in the portal tracts may result in portal hypertension. The extensive portal fibrosis and obliteration of the portal veins in this patient was due to chronic inorganic *arsenic* ingestion. For many years he had received sodium arsenite (Fowler's solution) for the relief of psoriasis. A similar picture may be seen in workers exposed to *vinyl chloride monomers* which are used in the synthesis of the plastic P.V.C.

Extrahepatic portal hypertension

Thrombosis of the portal vein is the commonest cause of extrahepatic portal hypertension. This usually follows neonatal infection of the umbilicus. The infection spreads up the umbilical vein to the left branch of the portal vein and thence to the main portal vein causing thrombosis. Other causes include: intra-abdominal sepsis, such as appendicitis or a perforated duodenal ulcer, tumours of the pancreas and blood diseases with increased blood coagulation such as polycythaemia rubra vera.

301. Portal vein thrombosis following neonatal infection of the umbilicus. These children develop normally. Examination reveals an enlarged spleen as in this child. Splenomegaly often causes a pancytopenia. The liver is normal.

302. Portal vein thrombosis. Signs of previous umbilical infection may be present. This Arab child had extrahepatic portal vein thrombosis. This circular scar around the umbilicus results from native treatment at birth.

303. Enlarged spleen (arrowed) was visible in an x-ray of the abdomen in this patient with portal vein thrombosis. The liver was of normal size.

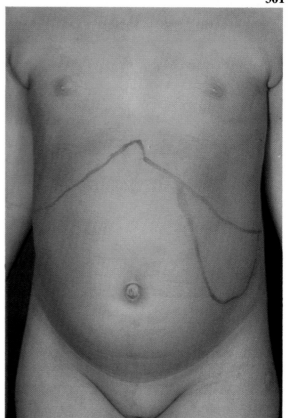

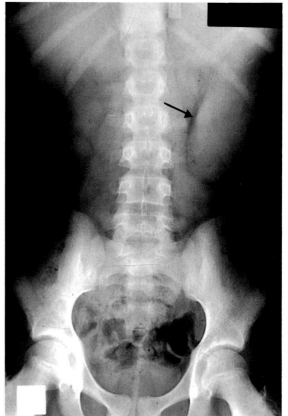

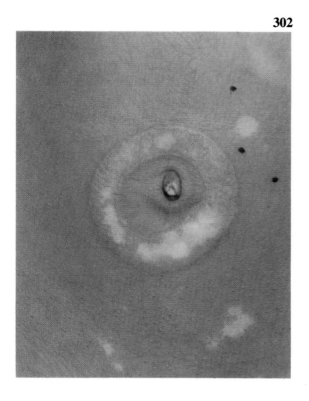

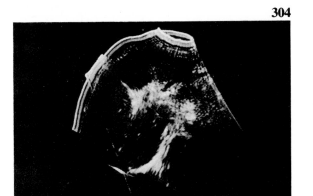
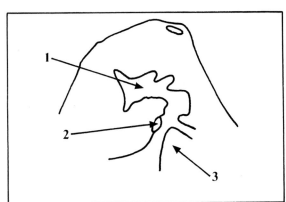

304. Grey scale ultrasonography will normally identify the portal vein in the porta hepatis (1). In portal vein thrombosis the portal vein is absent. In this scan the inferior vena cava (2) and a vertebral body (3) can also be seen.

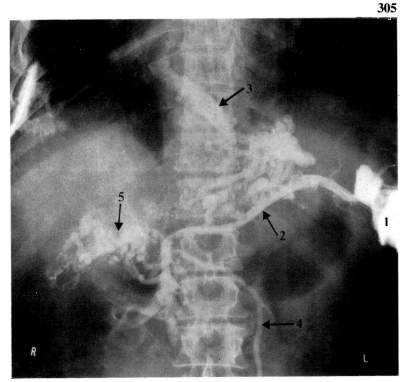

305. Splenic venogram in portal vein thrombosis. The splenic injection (1) filled the splenic vein (2) and collaterals to a mesh of oesophageal varices (3). There is retrograde flow down the inferior mesenteric vein (4). The portal vein had been replaced by many small collaterals (5). In this patient no cause was found for the portal vein thrombosis.

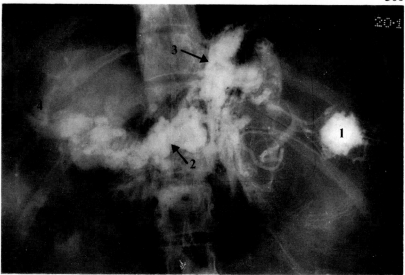

306. Splenic venogram in a patient with thrombosis of the splenic vein and portal vein. Injection of contrast into the splenic pulp (1) entered numerous collateral channels (2) shunting blood past the blocked splenic and portal veins. A leash of oesophageal varices (3) filled from the collaterals. Eventually some contrast filled the intrahepatic portal veins (4). This girl had had an umbilical infection soon after birth.

307

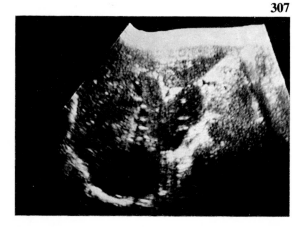 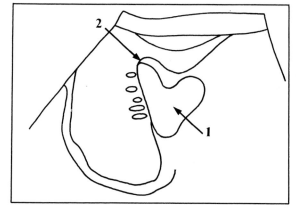

307. Cancer of the pancreas occasionally results in portal vein thrombosis. This 55-year-old man presented with bleeding oesophageal varices due to portal hypertension. An ultrasound scan showed a pancreatic mass (1) extending into the porta hepatis (2). The portal vein was not identified, suggesting portal vein obstruction.

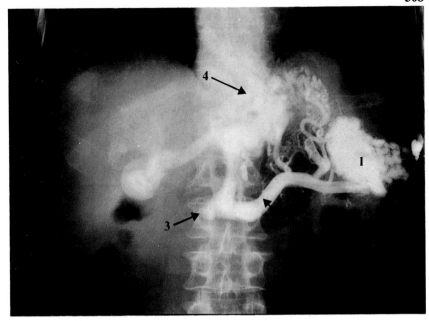

308. Cancer of the pancreas. A splenic venogram from the patient in **307** confirmed the portal vein thrombosis. Splenic injection of contrast (1) filled the splenic vein (2) which ended abruptly at the origin of the portal vein (3). Gastric and oesophageal varices (4) filled via collaterals from the splenic vein.

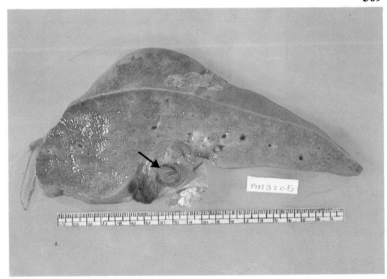

309. Cirrhosis is rare cause of portal vein thrombosis. A thrombosed portal vein (arrow) is visible at the porta hepatis in this section of a cirrhotic liver. Thrombosis of the portal vein is probably due to the sluggish portal circulation in cirrhosis. More commonly in cirrhotic patients, non-filling of the portal vein, during splenic venography, is due to diversion of blood down a large collateral circulation while the portal vein is in fact patent.

Hepatic artery

310. Hepatic artery occlusion leads to infarction of the liver. The pale infarcted areas are surrounded by red haemorrhagic zones. This rare condition may follow polyarteritis nodosa, emboli from bacterial endocarditis and biliary tract surgery. Hepatic artery occlusion is rarely diagnosed during life.

310

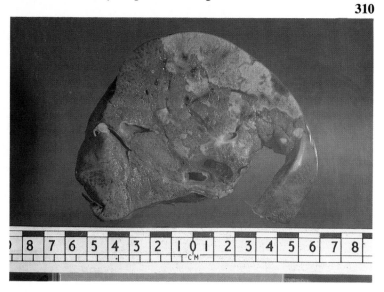

311

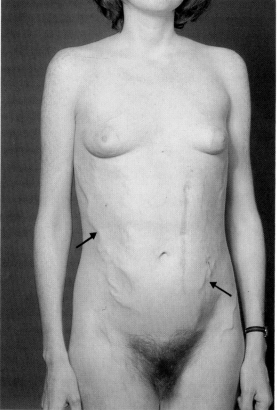

Hepatic veins

The hepatic veins drain into the inferior vena cava where it passes through the liver. The number of hepatic veins is variable. In general, one vein drains the left lobe and two veins drain the right lobe. The caudate lobe of the liver is drained separately into the inferior vena cava by a variable number of small veins.

311. Hepatic venous obstruction (Budd-Chiari syndrome). In the acute type the patient usually dies in liver failure. More commonly, a chronic form is encountered as in this patient. The liver was enlarged and tender. Obstruction of the inferior vena cava caused the dilated veins on her abdominal wall (arrowed) and oedema of the legs. The flow of blood in these veins was upwards. In this patient the hepatic vein obstruction was associated with the oral contraceptive pill. Other causes include: congenital webs, clotting diseases, thrombosis of the inferior vena cava due to renal or adrenal carcinomas, veno-occlusive disease, acute alcoholic hepatitis and constrictive pericarditis.

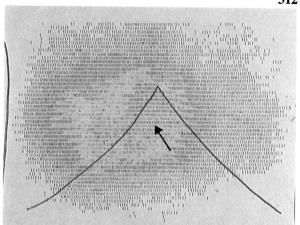

312. Isotope scan may be characteristic in hepatic venous obstruction. There is reduced uptake of ^{99}technetium by the areas of the liver with an obstructed venous drainage. However, the caudate lobe, which has a separate venous drainage, is relatively spared. The caudate lobe may hypertrophy, resulting in excessive isotope uptake. This scan shows a central 'hot' area (arrow) due to the caudate lobe surrounded by poor uptake in the rest of the liver.

313

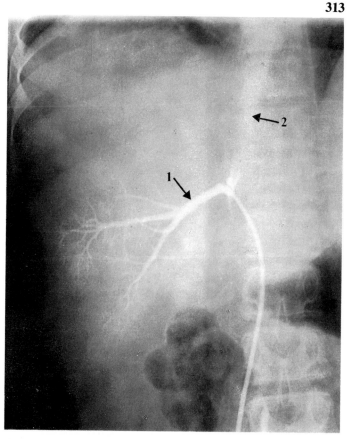

313. Hepatic venography. Cannulation of the hepatic veins through the superior or inferior vena cava is essential to determine the site of the hepatic vein block. This x-ray shows the normal branching pattern in one of the right hepatic veins (1). Some contrast can be seen flowing up the vena cava (2).

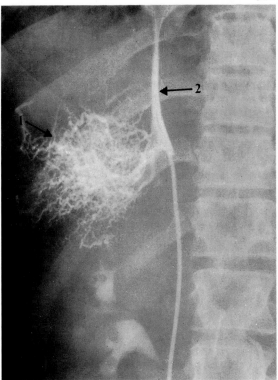

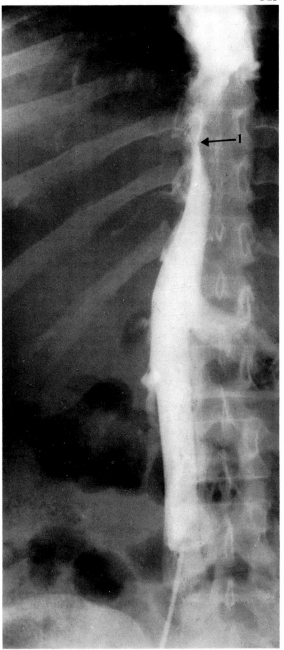

314. Hepatic venography in hepatic venous obstruction. The right hepatic vein has been cannulated via the inferior vena cava. The normal 'tree-like' pattern of the hepatic veins in the liver has been replaced by a characteristic 'lace-like' pattern (1). Contrast is escaping up the vena cava (2). In some patients extensive thrombosis in the hepatic veins will prevent cannulation. In this patient the Budd-Chiari syndrome followed trauma to the liver.

315. Inferior vena-cavography should also be performed in the Budd-Chiari syndrome. This usually reveals a narrowed segment (1) where the inferior vena cava passes through the liver due to compression by the hypertrophied caudate lobe. A supra-hepatic web obstructing the inferior vena cava may also be shown. Pressure measurements along the course of the inferior vena cava will establish the degree and site of obstruction due to a caudate lobe or vena-caval web.

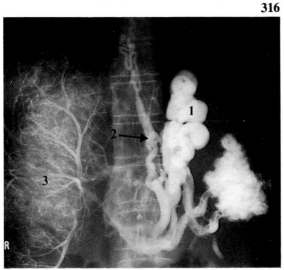

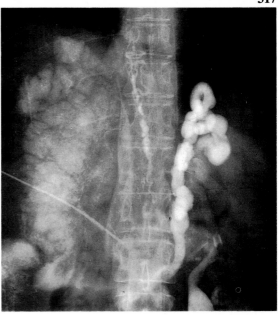

316. Portal hypertension develops in chronic hepatic venous obstruction. This splenic venogram shows an extensive collateral circulation arising from the splenic and portal veins. A large retroperitoneal collateral (1) and shunts to oesophageal varices (2) have filled. The liver is grossly enlarged (3) and there is 'pooling' of the contrast in the liver. The Budd-Chiari syndrome in this patient followed the oral contraceptive pill.

317. Transhepatic portal venogram in the patient shown in **316**. A later x-ray in this study shows circular collections of contrast in the enlarged liver. This appearance may be mistaken for malignant deposits in the liver.

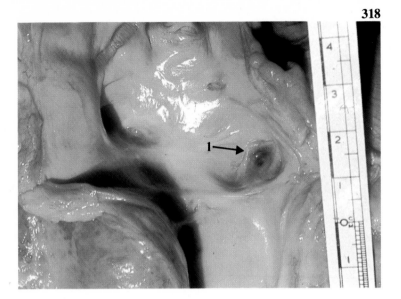

318. Hepatic venous obstruction. A thrombosed hepatic vein (1) is visible on laying open the intrahepatic portion of the inferior vena cava in this patient with the Budd-Chiari syndrome. However the obstruction may be at any point along the length of the hepatic veins.

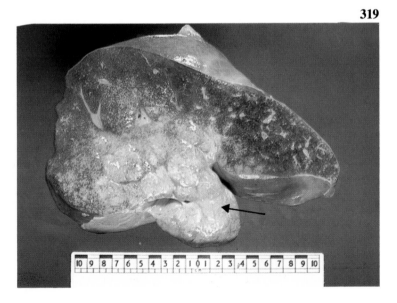

319. Hepatic venous obstruction. In this section of the liver at autopsy the dark areas are congested due to venous obstruction. The pale areas are regenerating liver tissue. Note the marked hypertrophy of the caudate lobe (arrow).

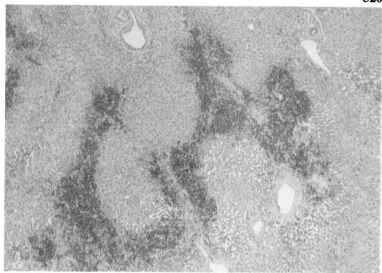

320. Hepatic venous obstruction. A liver biopsy is essential. This shows congestion and haemorrhage around the central veins. *(H. & E. ×10)*

Circulatory failure

A rise in right atrial pressure is readily transmitted to the hepatic veins. This results in impaired hepatic blood flow and oxygen supply especially to the centrizonal liver cells. Impaired tissue perfusion due to arterial hypotension further aggravates the oxygen supply to the hepatocytes in circulatory failure.

321

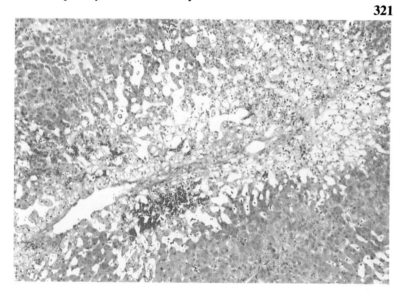

321. Acute heart failure. This biopsy came from a man who suffered a coronary thrombosis and prolonged hypotension. Around the central vein (which is stained blue) some liver cells have disappeared and others are necrotic. The sinusoids are dilated and there are areas of haemorrhage. The reticulin framework is preserved. These are the hepatic changes which develop in shock. *(Picro-Mallory×25)*

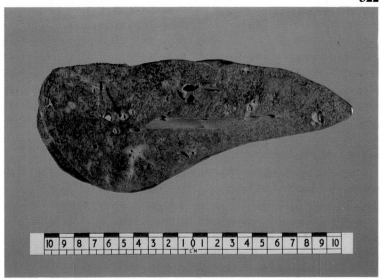

322. Congestive cardiac failure when prolonged gives a 'nutmeg' liver. The cut surface shows yellow areas caused by fatty peripheral zones alternating with red areas due to centrizonal congestion and haemorrhage. The hepatic veins (1) are prominent and their walls are thickened. Prolonged heart failure results in condensation of the centrizonal reticulin and later fibrous bands link the central veins. Finally, a cardiac cirrhosis may develop.

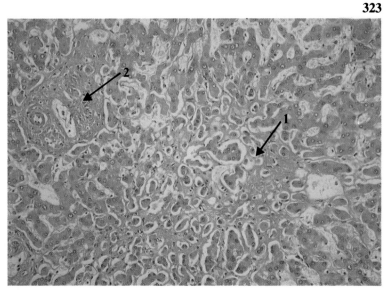

323. Congestive cardiac failure. Extensive fibrous tissue, stained pale blue, has developed around the central vein (1) in this patient with long-standing heart failure. Fibrous septa extend from the centrizonal areas to link the central veins. In chronic cases the portal tracts (2) are surrounded by a cuff of fibrous tissue. *(Martius-Scarlet-Blue×40)*

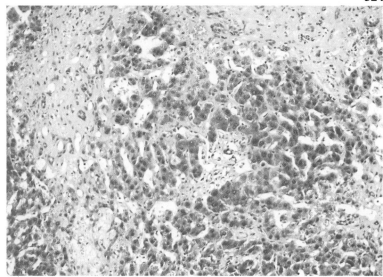

324. Cardiac cirrhosis. In prolonged heart failure centrizonal fibrosis increases and fibrous septa extend to link the central veins, isolating nodules of liver cells. In this severe case a cardiac cirrhosis has developed. *(H. & E. ×40)*

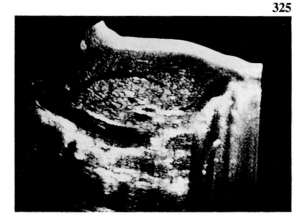

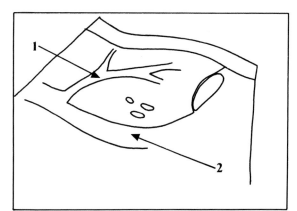

325. Congestive cardiac failure. Grey-scale ultrasonography shows dilatation of the hepatic veins (1) and inferior vena cava (2) in this patient with congestive cardiac failure. This is caused by transmission of the high right atrial pressure.

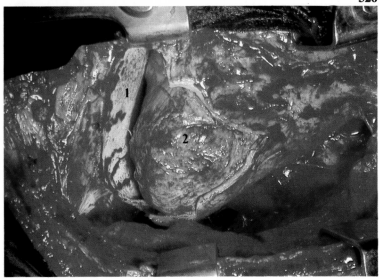

326. Constrictive pericarditis has a similar effect on the liver as congestive cardiac failure. Patients usually present with marked ascites and a hard, enlarged, non-pulsatile liver. Other features of constrictive pericarditis must be sought, including a paradoxical arterial pulse, the characteristic jugular venous pulse and a calcified pericardium. This patient was treated by stripping the tough fibrous pericardium (1) from the heart (2).

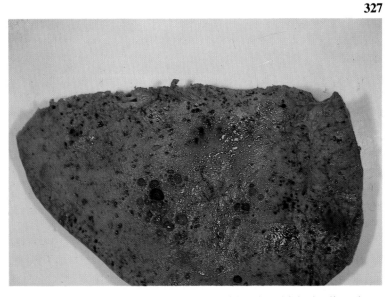

327. Peliosis hepatis is a very rare condition in which the liver has a bluish colour and contains numerous blue-black blood filled sacs. Rupture of the cysts may result in severe haemorrhage. The aetiology of peliosis hepatis is unknown but it is associated with fatal tuberculosis, anabolic steroids and oral contraceptives (see also Adenomas of the liver, Chapter 10).

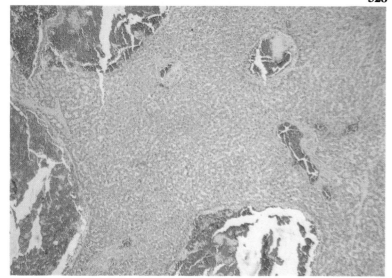

328. Peliosis hepatis. A liver biopsy shows normal liver tissue studded with large blood filled spaces. Some have no endothelial lining, while others are dilated sinusoids, portal or central veins. *(H. & E. ×10)*

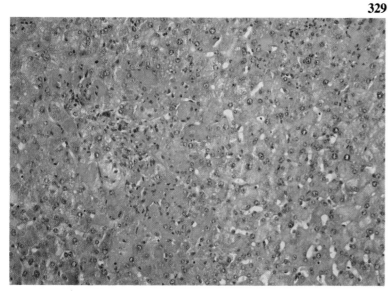

329. Eclampsia of pregnancy. Jaundice is terminal and usually follows the grand mal seizures. The liver shows extensive periportal pink staining fibrin deposition in the sinusoids. Centrizonal changes of necrosis and haemorrhage indicate shock. Characteristically there is no inflammatory reaction. This biopsy came from a 34-year-old woman. She was 36 weeks pregnant with twins when eclampsia suddenly developed. *(H. & E. ×40)*

7. *Storage diseases of the liver*

Iron storage diseases

These are classified as *haemochromatosis* where iron deposition has resulted in liver injury (usually cirrhosis) and *haemosiderosis* where there is excessive iron deposition in the liver but no tissue damage. Idiopathic (hereditary) haemochromatosis is due to increased intestinal absorption of iron. Rarely, secondary haemochromatosis develops after repeated transfusions, chronic haemolytic anaemia or excessive iron ingestion (Bantu siderosis).

330. Idiopathic haemochromatosis typically presents in middle-aged men. The patient is pigmented and body hair is scanty or absent. The liver is enlarged and the spleen may be palpable as in this patient. Diabetes mellitus is common.

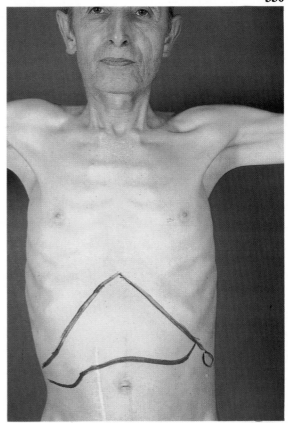

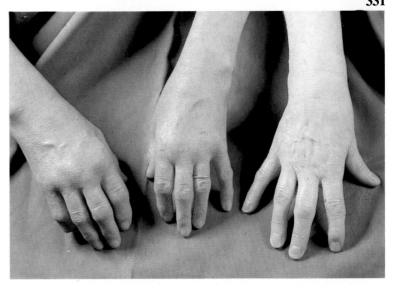

331. Idiopathic haemochromatosis. The skin pigmentation is a slate-grey colour and is due to increased melanin in the skin. It is maximal in the axillae, groins and exposed areas. The pigmented hands on the left come from a patient with haemochromatosis, the hand on the right is from an unaffected relative. Note the arthropathy affecting the first and second metacarpophalangeal joints.

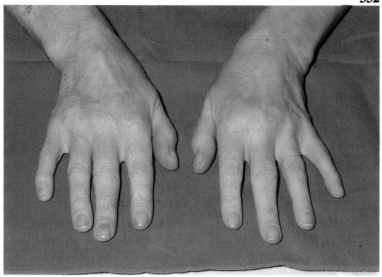

332. Idiopathic haemochromatosis. Many patients develop an arthropathy causing swelling of the first and second metacarpophalangeal joints. The arthritis is related to pyrophosphate crystal deposition. An x-ray of the hands may show chondrocalcinosis in the articular cartilage.

333

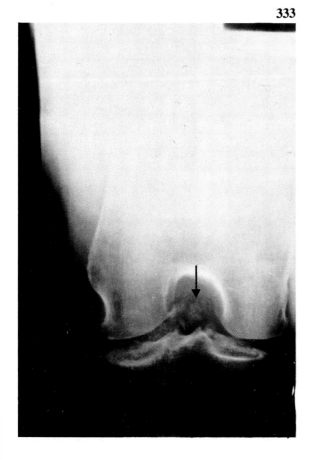

333. Idiopathic haemochromatosis. The pyrophosphate arthropathy also affects the knees. This x-ray of the knee in flexion shows chondrocalcinosis (arrowed) of the menisci and articular cartilage.

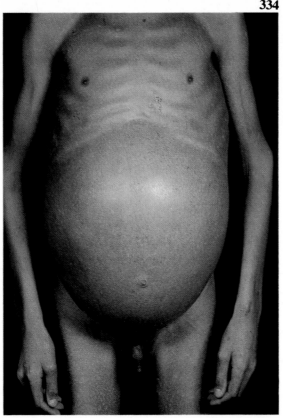

334. Idiopathic haemochromatosis. Primary liver cancer develops in some patients. Sudden clinical deterioration, with the development of ascites, often heralds a primary liver cancer, as in this patient. Note the pronounced skin pigmentation and muscle wasting.

335

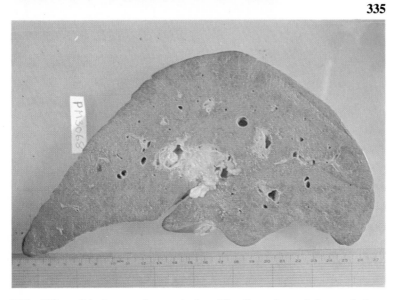

335. Idiopathic haemochromatosis. The liver is nodular and the iron deposition gives it a bronze-like colour. Ultimately a macronodular cirrhosis develops.

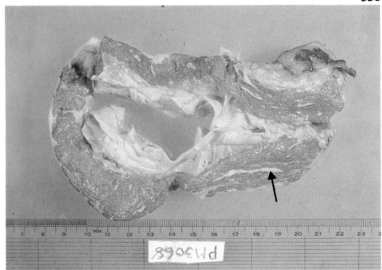

336. Idiopathic haemochromatosis. Iron deposited in the pancreas gives it a bronzed colour. This picture shows the pancreas laid open; the pancreatic duct is arrowed. The iron causes destruction of the pancreatic parenchyma and fibrosis. Diabetes mellitus is a common sequel. Bronze diabetes was an early name for idiopathic haemochromatosis.

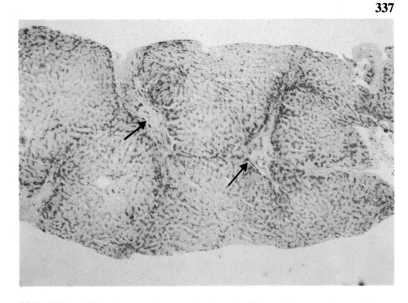

337. Idiopathic haemochromatosis. A liver biopsy shows iron (stained blue) deposited mainly in the liver cells but also in Kupffer cells. Most of the iron is concentrated around the portal tracts (arrow). Fibrous septa extend from the portal tracts giving a 'holly leaf' appearance. *(Perls ×16)*

338. Idiopathic haemochromatosis.
Stained with haematoxylin and eosin, the biopsy in **337** shows focal areas of inflammation and active fibrous septa around portal tracts. The brown material is iron. *(×16)*

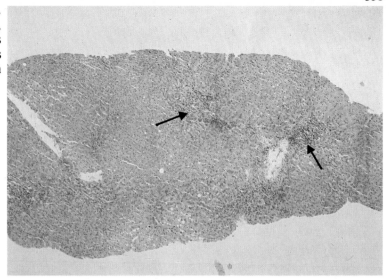

339. Idiopathic haemochromatosis.
Four years later, after repeated venesections, a further biopsy from the patient in **337** shows complete removal of iron from the liver. *(Perls ×16)*

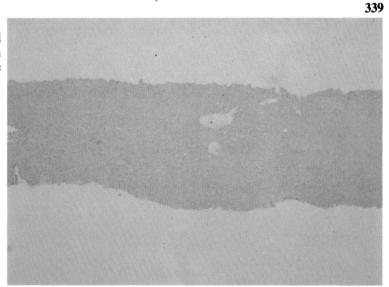

340. Idiopathic haemochromatosis.
A haematoxylin and eosin stain of the biopsy in **339** showed that, following the removal of iron, the liver histology had returned to normal.

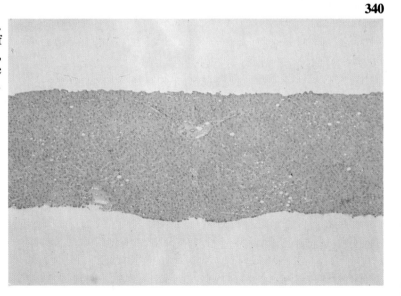

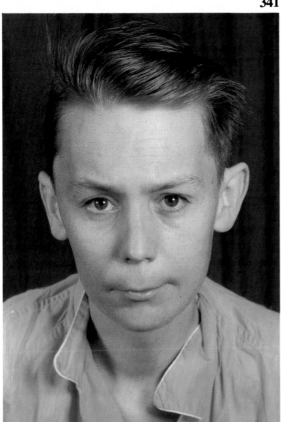

341. Secondary haemochromatosis. The slate-grey skin pigmentation can be seen on the face. A congenital haemolytic anaemia was the cause of iron overload in this young man.

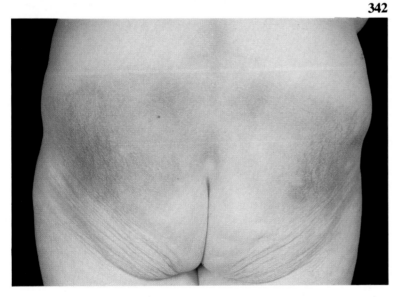

342. Secondary haemochromatosis. This patient had idiopathic sideroblastic anaemia. Iron absorption is increased because of the excessive erythropoietic activity. Iron overload caused the skin pigmentation on her buttocks and the hepatomegaly. Secondary iron overload is also seen in thalassaemia and sickle cell anaemia.

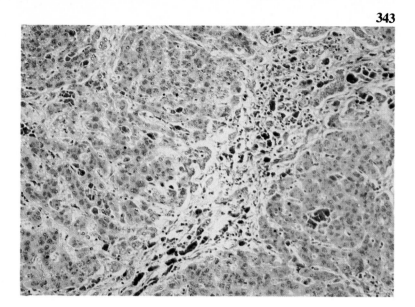

343. Secondary haemochromatosis. Cirrhosis had developed in the patient in **342**. Fibrous septa separate nodules of liver cells. The brown pigment represents iron deposits. *(H. & E. ×40)*

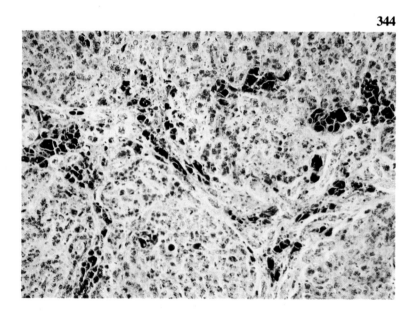

344. Secondary haemochromatosis. A Perls stain of the biopsy in **343** shows the widespread iron as blue staining material. Iron is first deposited in the Kupffer cells and later in the hepatocytes. *(×40)*

Wilson's disease (hepatolenticular degeneration)

This is a rare cause of inherited cirrhosis principally affecting children and young adults. It is characterised by cirrhosis, degeneration of the basal ganglia, renal tubular damage and brown rings in the cornea (Kayser-Fleischer rings). Copper accumulates in many organs.

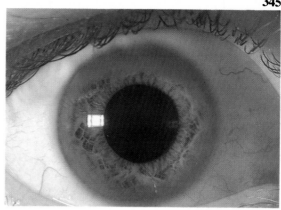

345

345. Kayser-Fleischer rings are greenish-brown rings at the periphery of the cornea. They are caused by the deposition of copper on the posterior surface of the cornea and appear first at the upper pole. Kayser-Fleischer rings are present in practically every symptomatic case of Wilson's disease but a slit lamp examination may be required to detect them.

346. Wilson's disease may present with an episode of jaundice due to haemolysis or as a well compensated cirrhosis. Alternatively Wilson's disease can mimic chronic active hepatitis, as in this young woman. Note the abdominal striae and leg oedema. The posture and fatuous expression in this patient are due to the basal ganglia changes of Wilson's disease, which usually develop some years after the liver disease.

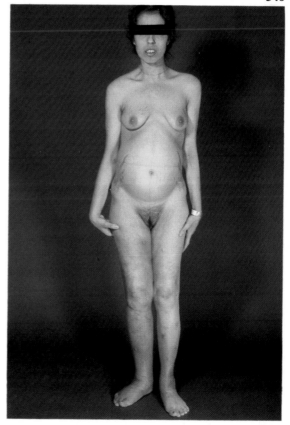

346

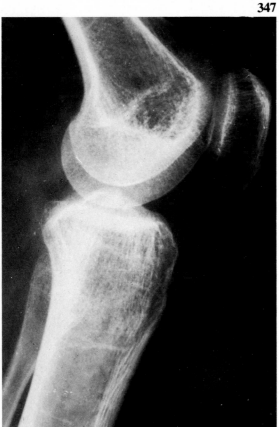

347. Wilson's disease. The bones may be demineralised. Sub-articular cysts and fragmentation of bone also develop. Note the demineralised femur and tibia in this patient.

348

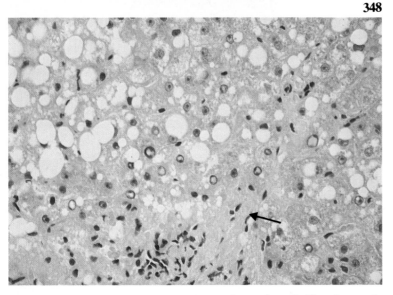

348. Wilson's disease. A liver biopsy shows fatty infiltration and vacuolated nuclei (glycogenic vacuolation). Some of the liver cells are ballooned and the inflammatory reaction is usually slight. A fibrous septum is present (arrow). *(H.&E. ×100)*

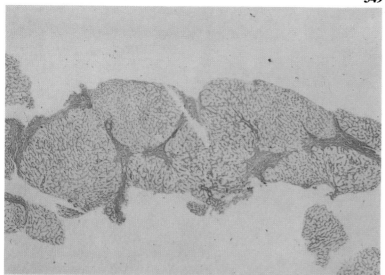

349. Wilson's disease. A reticulin stain of the biopsy showed cirrhosis with fibrous septa separating nodules of varying sizes. Cirrhosis is usual in symptomatic patients. *(×10)*

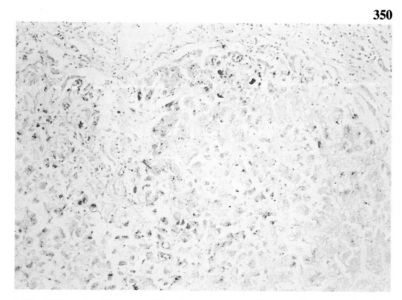

350. Wilson's disease. The large accumulation of copper in the liver cells has been stained reddish-pink in this biopsy. Histological stains for copper are unreliable for the diagnosis of Wilson's disease. *(Rhodanine ×40)*

Alpha₁ anti-trypsin deficiency

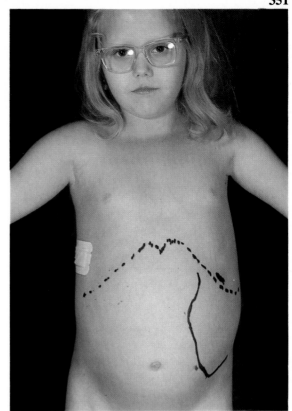

This inherited metabolic defect is associated with neonatal hepatitis and cirrhosis in children and pulmonary emphysema in adults. In most patients the cholestatic neonatal hepatitis subsides by about seven months but later hepatosplenomegaly develops due to a cirrhosis. However, the presentation of alpha₁ anti-trypsin deficiency is variable and rarely patients present with cirrhosis in later life. The serum alpha₁ anti-trypsin concentration is low.

351. Alpha₁ anti-trypsin deficiency. This girl had neonatal hepatitis. Aged five, cirrhosis was present with splenomegaly due to portal hypertension. Now, aged nine, she suffered repeated haematemeses from oesophageal varices. Her brother also had alpha₁ anti-trypsin deficiency.

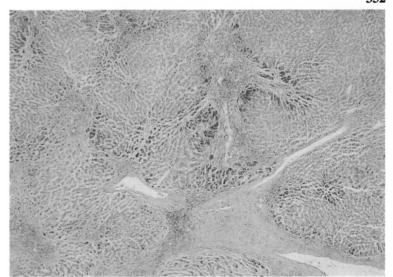

352. Alpha₁ anti-trypsin deficiency. A liver biopsy showed a cirrhotic liver with brightly staining diastase resistant inclusions concentrated around the portal tracts. *(Diastase periodic acid Schiff×10)*

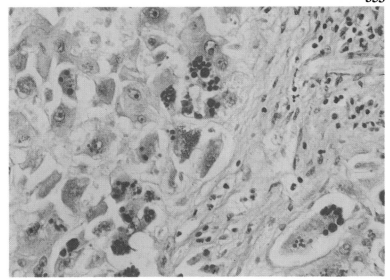

353. Alpha₁ anti-trypsin deficiency. At a higher magnification the bright red granular inclusions are seen to be in the liver cells around the portal tracts. *(Diastase periodic acid Schiff × 100)*

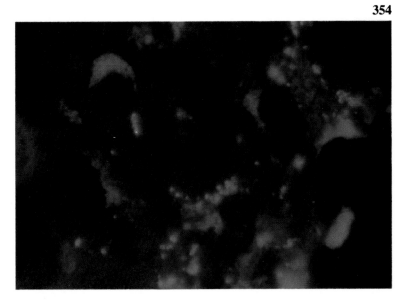

354. Alpha₁ anti-trypsin deficiency. This biopsy has been stained specifically with a fluorescent bound antibody to alpha₁ anti-trypsin. The blue granules represent accumulation of alpha₁ anti-trypsin in the liver cells. *(× 400)*

Fatty infiltration

Infiltration of the liver with fat occurs in a variety of common conditions including obesity, alcoholism and diabetes mellitus. Rare causes of massive fatty change are acute fatty liver of pregnancy and, in children, Reye's syndrome (fatty change with encephalopathy).

355

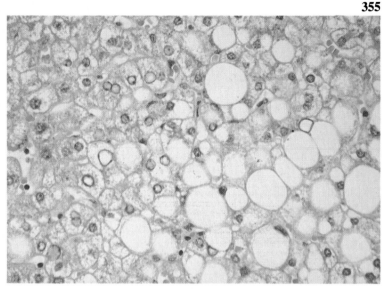

355. Fatty liver. Many liver cells are distended with fat droplets and the nuclei are vacuolated. The fatty change is most marked around the portal zones. During the processing of the section the fat droplets were dissolved, leaving empty spaces. This biopsy came from a diabetic patient. *(H.&E.×100)*

356

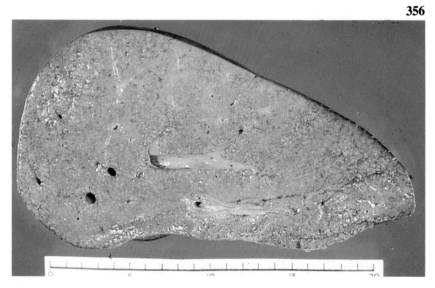

356. Fatty liver. The liver is enlarged and light coloured. The cut surface is greasy and reveals yellow areas of periportal fat. This is the liver of an alcoholic.

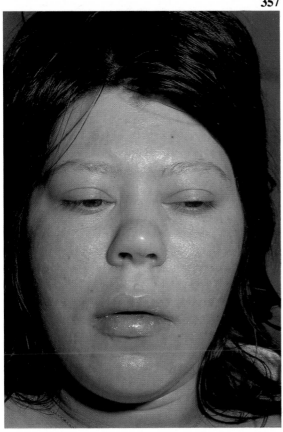

357. Acute fatty liver of pregnancy is a rare cause of jaundice and liver failure in pregnancy. This 23-year-old primiparous patient developed vomiting and epigastric pain followed by jaundice, hepatic encephalopathy and anuria when 37 weeks pregnant.

358

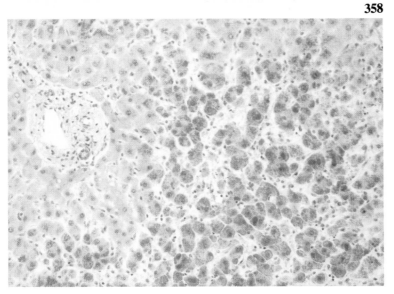

358. Acute fatty liver of pregnancy. A liver biopsy is diagnostic. The liver is massively infiltrated with fat droplets especially in the centrizonal areas. Liver cell necrosis and inflammation are insignificant. This biopsy has been processed to preserve the fat droplets which are stained red. *(Oil red 0×40)*

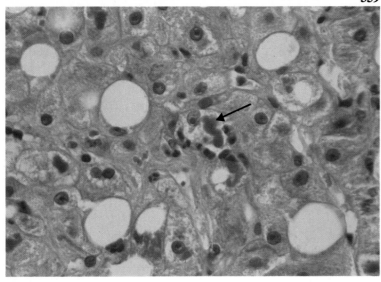

359. Jejuno-ileal bypass may cause liver lesions indistinguishable from alcoholic hepatitis. This biopsy shows fat droplets and alcoholic hyaline (arrowed) surrounded by a cuff of polymorphonuclear leucocytes. The patient was a 30-year-old American woman from the 'Bible belt' who had never tasted alcohol. *(Mallory ×100)*

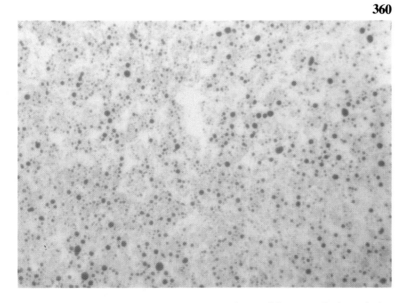

360. Reye's syndrome (fatty infiltration with encephalopathy) affects children under 10 years of age. Following an upper respiratory infection, this four-year-old boy developed seizures and coma. The prothrombin time was prolonged 4 seconds over the control value and the arterial ammonia concentration was raised. Hypoglycaemia and intracranial hypertension are frequent complications. The liver biopsy shows massive infiltration with fine droplet fat (stained red). *(Oil Red 0×200)*

Glycogen storage diseases

There are many varieties of these inherited defects of glycogen metabolism. The severity and prognosis of the disease depends on the type. Typically, patients present in childhood with hepatomegaly and episodes of hypoglycaemia and ketosis.

361. Glycogen storage disease. This two-year-old child presented with massive hepatomegaly but characteristically the spleen was not enlarged. Although reduced in height, his weight was normal for his age.

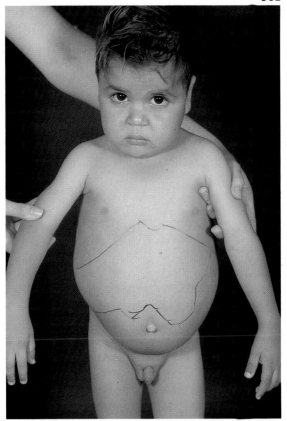

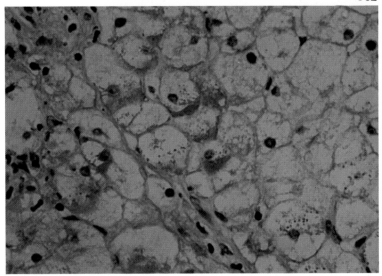

362. Glycogen storage disease. A liver biopsy shows swollen liver cells and vacuolated nuclei full of glycogen. Enzyme analysis of the liver biopsy will determine the type of glycogen storage disease. *(Periodic acid Schiff × 100)*

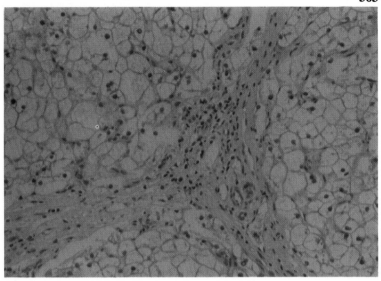

363. Glycogen storage disease. In a liver biopsy processed in formol saline the glycogen is washed out of the cells. The liver cells then appear clear like plant cells. *(H. & E. × 40)*

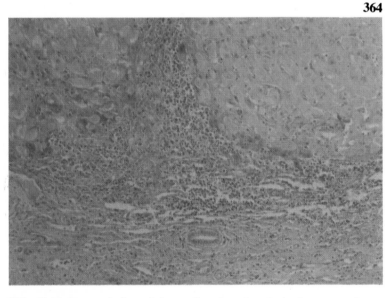

364. Galactosaemia is an inborn disorder of carbohydrate metabolism. Galactose-1-phosphate accumulates, derived mainly from dietary milk. Infants present with diarrhoea, vomiting and frequently jaundice. A macronodular cirrhosis and cataracts develop. This biopsy shows an enlarged fibrotic portal tract containing inflammatory cells surrounded by regenerative nodules. Giant cells and pseudo-acini may be prominent. *(Periodic acid Schiff × 40)*

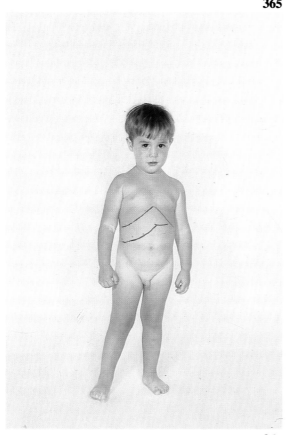

365. Hereditary fructose intolerance. This 2½-year-old boy presented with nausea, vomiting and hepatomegaly. Hypoglycaemia, jaundice and aminoaciduria may also develop. Fructose intolerance resembles galactosaemia but the presentation is usually delayed until fruit and sucrose are introduced to the diet.

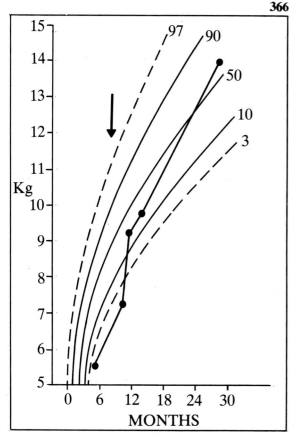

366. Hereditary fructose intolerance. Development is retarded. At presentation this child's weight was below the third percentile. After removal of fructose and sucrose from his diet, his weight rapidly returned to normal.

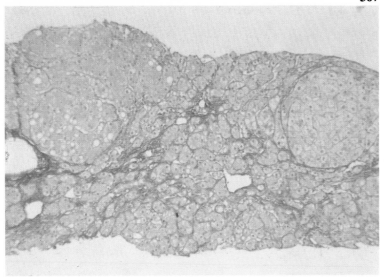

367. Hereditary fructose intolerance. In the liver fatty infiltration, liver cell necrosis, fibrosis and bile ductular proliferation develop. In this patient prolonged fructose ingestion had led to cirrhosis. *(×16)*

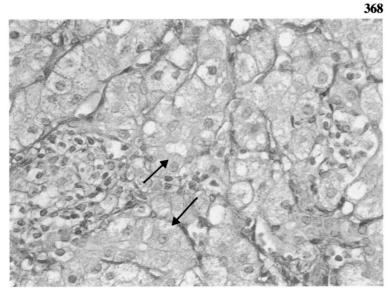

368. Hereditary fructose intolerance. A higher magnification of the biopsy in **367** shows chronic inflammatory cell infiltration, fatty change and fibrosis. Groups of liver cells forming pseudo-acini (arrowed) are prominent. *(×100)*

Lipid storage diseases

369. Familial hypercholesterolaemia. The hetero-zygote develops skin xanthomas and ischaemic heart disease in middle age. The homozygous state is rare and presents in childhood. The development of this five-year-old homozygote girl was normal when she presented with skin xanthomas. Her serum cholesterol level was 420mg/100ml.

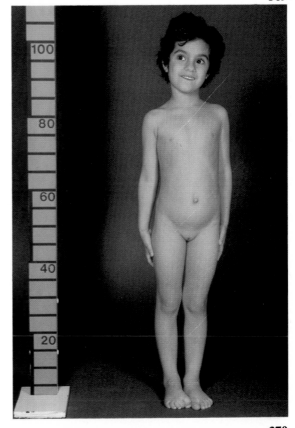

370. Familial hypercholesterolaemia. Tuberous xanthomas had developed on the hands of the patient shown in **369**. Tendon xanthomas were also present.

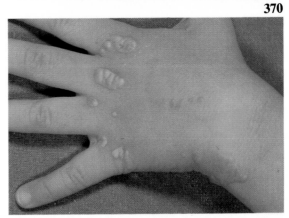

371. Familial hypercholesterolaemia. The white band at the upper pole of the cornea in the child shown in **369** is an arcus senilis, reflecting the high serum cholesterol concentration.

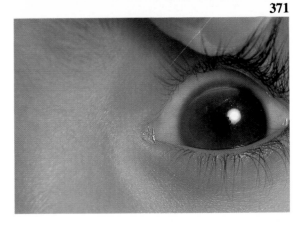

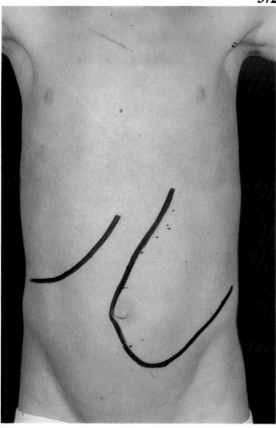

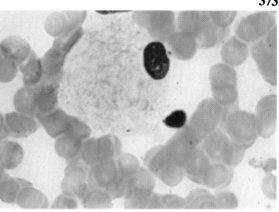

373. Gaucher's disease. A bone marrow aspirate may reveal the characteristic Gaucher cells. These are large, pale staining oval or polygonal cells 70–80μ in diameter. The cytoplasm is fibrillary and contains one or more hyperchromatic nuclei. *(May-Grünwald-Giemsa × 600)*

372. Gaucher's disease. In this rare inherited metabolic defect, a cerebroside accumulates in the reticulo-endothelial cells. The affected children present with hepato-splenomegaly. A chronic adult form of Gaucher's disease is more commonly encountered.

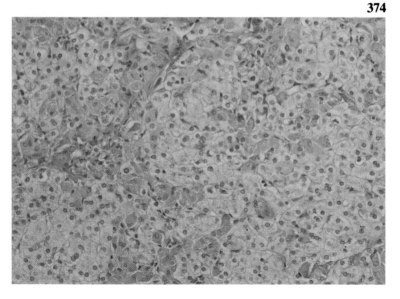

374. Gaucher's disease. A liver biopsy reveals heavy infiltration of pink staining Gaucher cells among the pale staining liver cells. *(Diastase periodic acid Schiff × 63)*

375. Gaucher's disease. At a higher magnification, the whole field is occupied by large pale staining Gaucher cells in this liver biopsy. *(H. & E. ×254)*

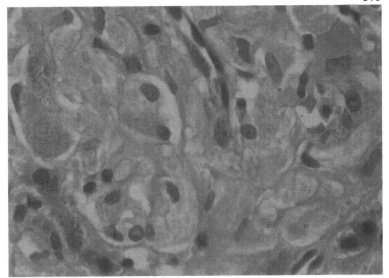

375a

375a. Niemann-Pick disease is a rare familial lipid storage disorder. Sphingomyelin accumulates in the reticulo-endothelial cells. The disease affects infants who die before two years of age. Hepato-splenomegaly and lymph node enlargement develop. The skin becomes waxy and yellow-brown. A cherry red spot may be seen at the macula of the ocular fundus (also seen in Tay Sach's disease). This liver biopsy from a one-year-old child shows the characteristic pale, swollen reticulo-endothelial cells packed with sphingomyelin (1). The liver cells are stained pink due to glycogen but also contain fine vacuoles of sphingomyelin (2). *(Periodic acid Schiff ×100)*

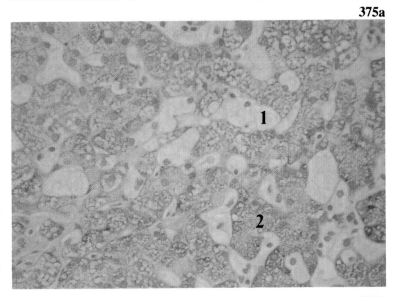

375a

375b. Niemann-Pick disease. An electronmicrograph of the biopsy in **375a** shows a liver cell (1) and two non-parenchymal cells (2). The cells are loaded with vacuoles (cytosomes) containing concentrically laminated material. This is sphingomyelin. *(×1900)*

375b

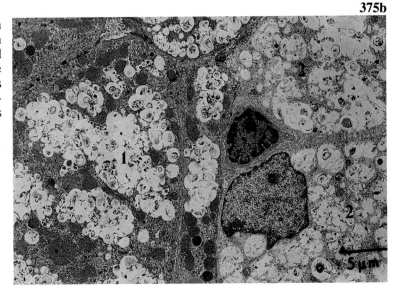

Amyloidosis

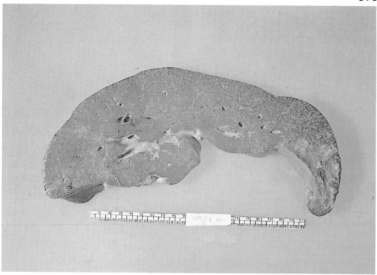

376. Amyloid infiltration of the liver leads to hepatomegaly. The cut surface has a firm, waxy texture. The amyloid deposits have been stained a reddish-brown colour with a dilute iodine solution. Staining with congo red is specific for amyloid. This patient developed amyloidosis following long-standing rheumatoid arthritis. Amyloidosis of the liver may complicate many other chronic diseases including tuberculosis, leprosy, pulmonary suppuration, ulcerative colitis, Crohn's disease, multiple myeloma and Hodgkin's disease. Primary amyloidosis (pericollagen or atypical) is a further rare form.

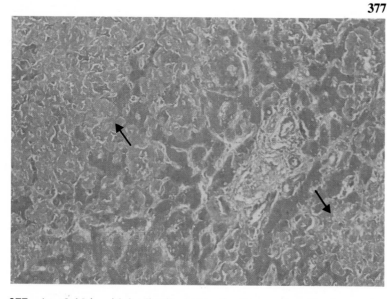

377. Amyloid is widely distributed in the liver and easily detected in a liver biopsy. The amorphous, dark staining amyloid is deposited between the liver cells and the sinusoidal wall in the Space of Disse (arrowed). *(Methyl violet×40)*

Cystic fibrosis (mucoviscidosis)

The commonest effects of this recessively inherited disorder are pancreatic insufficiency and recurrent chest infections. Cystic fibrosis may also involve the liver causing fatty change and a characteristic biliary cirrhosis.

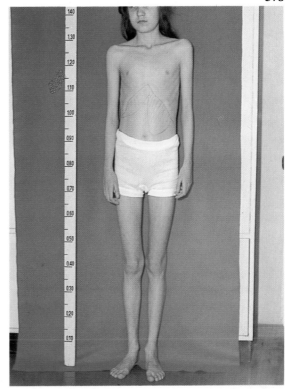

378. Cystic fibrosis in a 13-year-old girl. Biliary cirrhosis and portal venous hypertension have caused hepatosplenomegaly. Note the muscle wasting and barrel-shaped chest.

379. Cystic fibrosis. Peritoneoscopy in a seven-year-old boy with biliary cirrhosis and portal hypertension. A portal-systemic collateral vein is coursing over the surface of the nodular liver.

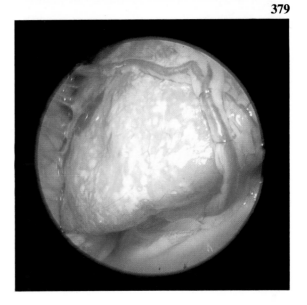

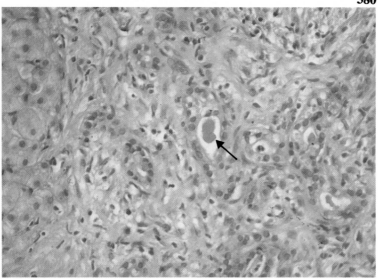

380. Cystic fibrosis. A liver biopsy from the boy in **379** shows a portal tract expanded by fibrosis and dilated proliferating bile ducts. The cast of eosinophilic material (arrowed) obstructing an intra-hepatic bile duct is the typical finding in cystic fibrosis. Fibrous septa radiate from the portal tracts and result in a coarse biliary cirrhosis. *(H. &E. ×175)*

Porphyria

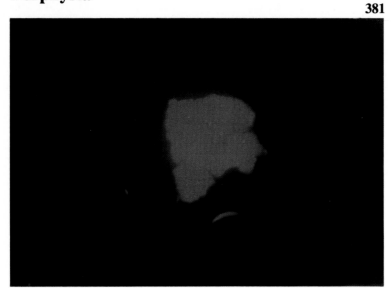

381. Porphyria cutanea tarda (symptomatic cutaneous hepatic porphyria). Uroporphyrin in a fresh fragment of liver biopsy gives a red fluorescence in ultra-violet light. Light microscopy shows a hepatitis or cirrhosis and iron overload. Symptoms include photosensitivity with blistering and scarring of the skin. Alcoholism is a common association. Urinary uroporphyrin excretion is increased.

8. Infections of the liver

Pyogenic infections

Pyogenic infections of the liver usually arise from the biliary tract (*cholangitis*) or the portal venous system (*portal pyaemia*). Stones or strictures in the biliary tract are the commonest causes of cholangitis. Portal pyaemia may follow intra-abdominal sepsis such as appendicitis, diverticulitis or a perforated duodenal ulcer. Both cholangitis and portal pyaemia may lead to a *pyogenic liver abscess*. Liver abscesses may rarely arise from the hepatic artery in the course of a *septicaemia*. In a proportion of patients no cause for the liver abscess can be found; these are termed '*cryptogenic*'. Organisms of the gut flora are usually cultured in these infections including the aerobes, such as *E. coli, str. faecalis, pr. vulgaris* and staphylococci and anaerobes such as bacteroides, aerobacter and anaerobic streptococci.

382. Recurrent cholangitis. This patient presented with recurrent rigors, sweating and fevers. He was not jaundiced. During the rigors, the white blood count rose to 18,000/mm³ and were mainly polymorphonuclear leucocytes. *E. coli* was cultured from his blood. This endoscopic retrograde cholangiogram showed a grossly dilated biliary tree with two large gallstones obstructing the lower end of the bile duct.

382

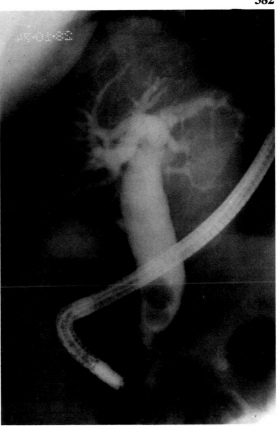

383

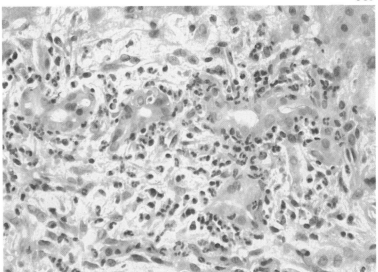

383. Recurrent cholangitis. A liver biopsy from the patient in **382** shows a severe cholangitis in the portal tracts. There is proliferation of the bile ductules and a heavy infiltrate of acute inflammatory cells. Culture of this biopsy yielded *E. coli*. *(H. & E. × 100)*

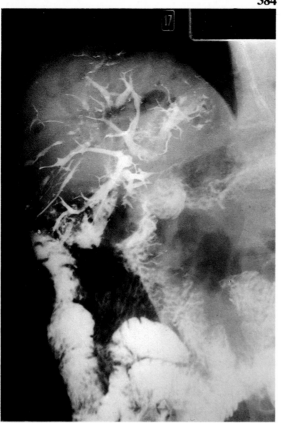

384. Recurrent cholangitis may follow surgical operations which permit reflux of the gut contents up the bile ducts. Following a choledocho-jejunostomy this patient had many attacks of cholangitis. A barium meal examination showed free reflux of the barium from the jejunum into the biliary tree. The small intrahepatic bile ducts, outlined by barium, showed the changes of secondary sclerosing cholangitis had followed the recurrent infections.

385

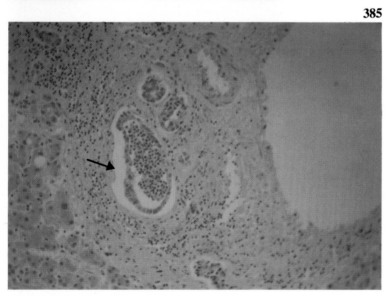

385. Suppurative cholangitis. A liver biopsy shows an enlarged portal zone massively infiltrated with acute inflammatory cells. A bile duct (arrowed) is full of pus. Culture of this biopsy yielded *E. coli. (H. & E. ×64)*

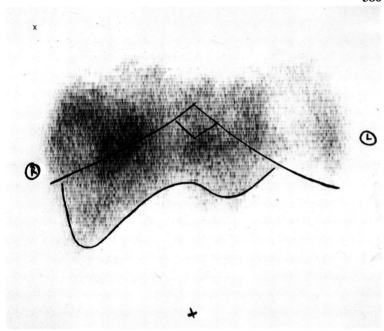

386. Pyogenic liver abscesses developed in this patient with gallstones obstructing the common bile duct. A ^{99}technetium isotope scan showed an enlarged liver containing multiple filling defects. Liver abscesses following cholangitis are commonly multiple.

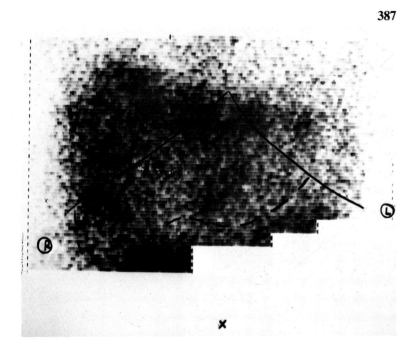

387. Pyogenic liver abscesses. A ^{67}gallium scan of the patient in **386** showed that the filling defects took up this isotope. ^{67}Gallium is taken up by the granulocytes in the walls of abscesses.

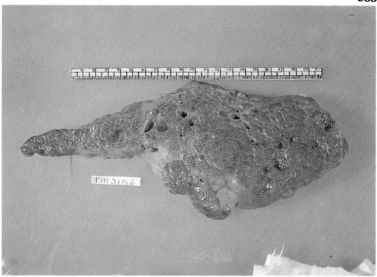

388. Pyogenic liver abscesses following acute suppurative cholangitis. A cut section of the liver shows multiple abscess cavities, about 1cm in diameter.

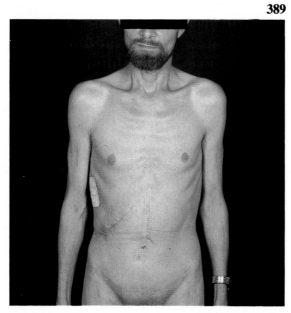

389. Pyogenic liver abscess following portal pyaemia. This patient developed rigors and a tender liver 10 days after a partial gastrectomy. Note the marked muscle wasting.

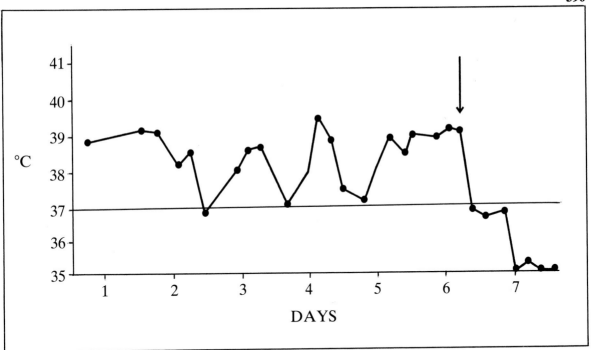

390. Pyogenic liver abscess. The temperature chart of the patient in **389** showed recurrent fevers up to 39.5°C. After surgical drainage of the abscess (arrowed) the temperature rapidly fell to normal.

391

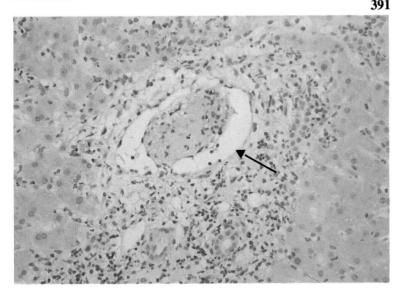

391. Pyogenic liver abscess. A liver biopsy from the patient in **389** showed pylephlebitis (septic phlebitis) of the portal vein. The portal tract is enlarged and contains an acute inflammatory infiltrate around the portal vein (arrowed). There is a thrombus in the portal vein. Portal vein thrombosis is a late complication of pylephlebitis. *(H. & E. ×63)*

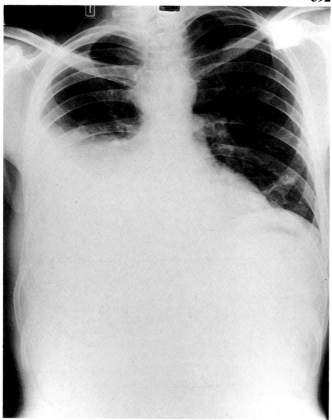

392. Pyogenic liver abscess. A chest x-ray of the patient in **389** showed a right-sided pleural effusion and a pulmonary reaction. This is a common finding with a liver abscess or sub-phrenic abscess.

393

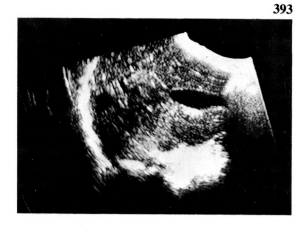 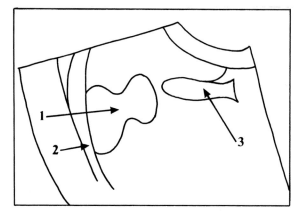

393. Grey-scale ultrasonography of the patient in **389**. A single abscess (1) was present lying posteriorly against the diaphragm (2). A normal gall bladder can also be seen (3).

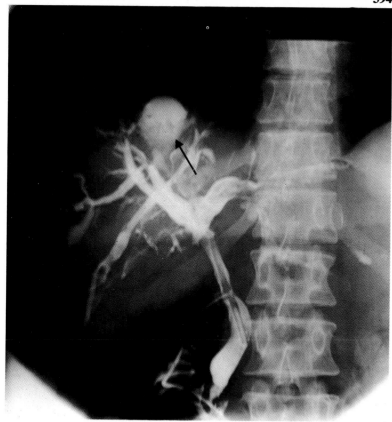

394. Pyogenic liver abscess. The abscess (arrowed) in the patient shown in **389** had involved the biliary tree and filled with contrast in a T-tube cholangiogram.

Amoebiasis of the liver

The protozoan parasite *Entamoeba histolytica* normally lives in the wall of the colon where it exists in two forms, a motile trophozoite and a non-motile cyst. The motile trophozoite invades the colonic mucosa where it may cause a colitis or enter the portal venous system and be carried to the liver. In the liver, *E. histolytica* secrete proteolytic enzymes which lyse liver tissue, resulting in abscess formation. These abscesses may burst into the pleural or peritoneal cavities. Amoebiasis is distributed throughout the world, but most infections are seen in the tropics.

395. Amoebic liver abscess. The patient is typically a young adult male. The liver may be enlarged and tender. An amoebic liver abscess is usually single and commonly found supero-anteriorly in the right lobe. Palpation may reveal an area of exquisite tenderness in the intercostal space overlying the abscess ('punch tenderness'). In this patient the tender point has been marked with a cross. A moderate polymorphonuclear leucocytosis develops. Only a small proportion of patients give a history of amoebic dysentery.

395

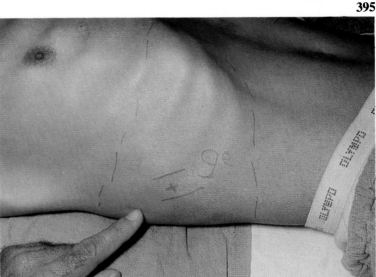

396

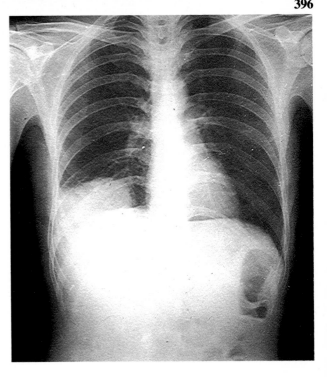

396. Amoebic liver abscess. A chest x-ray may show an elevated right hemidiaphragm as in this patient. In addition, a pleural effusion and a pulmonary reaction have developed.

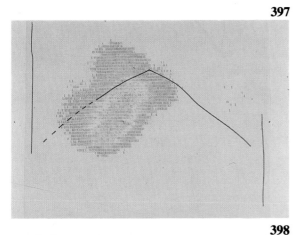

397

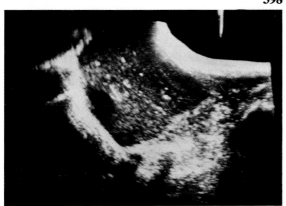

398

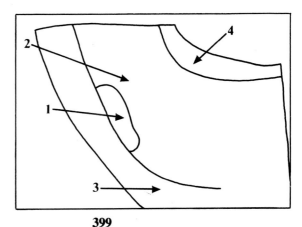

399

397. Amoebic liver abscess. A [99]technetium isotope scan is valuable in localising the site of the abscess. In this patient a filling defect due to an amoebic abscess is present in the superior part of the right lobe of the liver.

398. Amoebic liver abscess. A grey-scale ultrasonogram demonstrated an amoebic abscess (1) in the liver (2) lying posteriorly against the diaphragm (3). The anterior abdominal wall (4) is also shown. (Scanned 10cm right of the umbilicus).

399. Amoebic liver abscess in the right lobe of the liver displaced and stretched the intrahepatic vessels (arrowed) in this selective coeliac axis arteriogram.

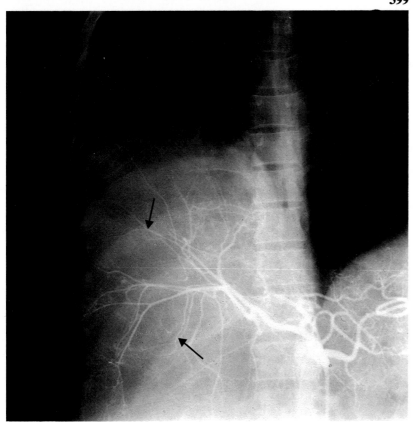

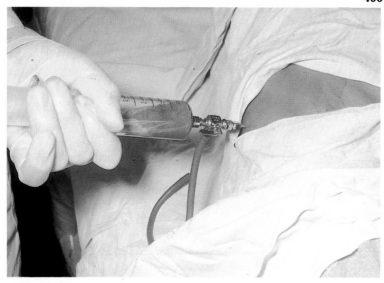

400. Amoebic liver abscess. Percutaneous drainage of an amoebic abscess yields reddish-brown pus ('anchovy sauce' or 'chocolate sauce'). The 'pus' consists of amoebae, degenerate and lysed liver cells and red blood cells. Secondary infection of the abscess occurs in a proportion of patients and the pus turns yellow or green and foul smelling.

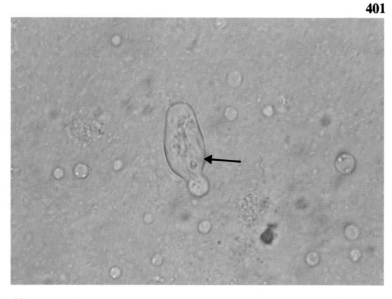

401. Amoebic liver abscess. A motile amoeba was found in the pus aspirated from the patient in **400** confirming the diagnosis.

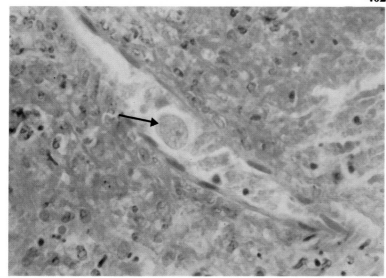

402. Amoebic liver abscess. The liver around the amoebic abscess shows necrotic liver cells. An amoeba (arrow) is present in a small portal vein radicle. *(H.&E.×100)*

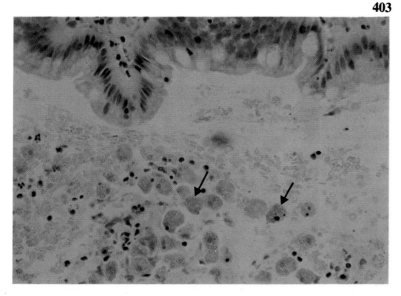

403. Amoebic colitis. Sigmoidoscopy and examination of fresh warm stools are essential in patients with a suspected amoebic abscess. In this patient an active amoebic colitis was seen and the rectal biopsy showed many motile amoebae (arrowed). The amoebae contain ingested red blood cells identifying them as *E. histolytica*. This is rare. Usually amoebic abscesses are not found in association with a very active colitis.

Hydatid disease

The tapeworm *Echinococcus granulosus* lives in the intestines of dogs. The ova shed by the tapeworm develop into cysts in the intermediate hosts: man, sheep and cattle. Dogs become infected by eating infected offal from sheep or cattle. Man is infected by contamination with dog faeces containing the ova. The ingested ova burrow through the intestinal wall and gain access to the liver via the portal venous system. In the liver the ova develop into hydatid cysts. Daughter cysts develop from the germinal layer of the wall of the hydatid cyst. Rarely, ova reach the systemic circulation and hydatid cysts develop in the lungs, spleen, brain and bone.

404. Hydatid cysts usually present with symptomless hepatomegaly as in this man. Some patients complain of a dull ache or distension in the right upper quadrant. Note the healthy appearance of the patient. Complications include secondary infection of the cyst and rupture of the cyst into the peritoneal or pleural cavities or the biliary system.

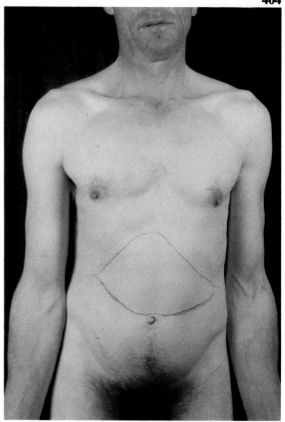

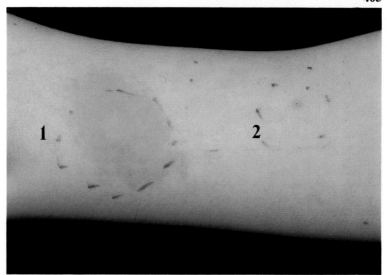

405. Casoni test. An intradermal injection of sterile hydatid cyst fluid (1) produces a wheal and flare after 12 hours in most patients with hydatid cysts. This is due to sensitisation of the patient by the specific hydatid antigens in the cyst fluid. Sterile saline (2) has also been injected as a control.

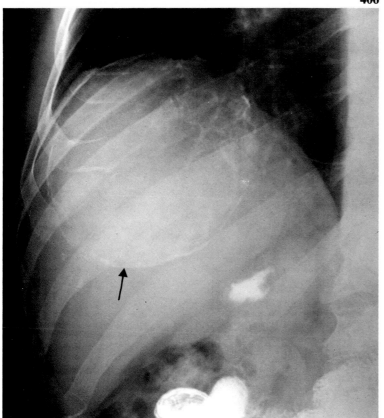

406. Hydatid cyst. An x-ray of the abdomen may show calcification in the wall of the cyst. In this patient the thin calcified wall reveals a large hydatid cyst in the right lobe of the liver under the diaphragm (arrowed).

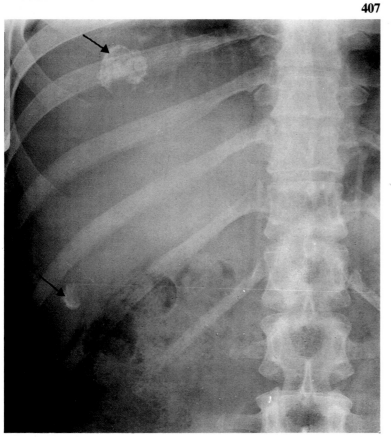

407. Hydatid cyst. In some patients the parasites die and the cysts degenerate and shrink. The calcium deposits in the cyst wall then appear like crumpled eggshells. Two dead hydatid cysts are present in this x-ray (arrowed).

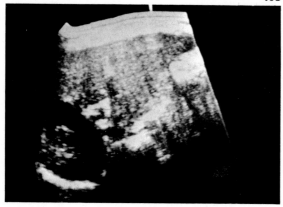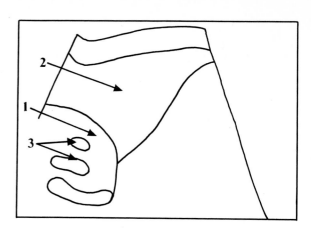

408. Hydatid cysts. To detect uncalcified cysts other techniques are used. This grey-scale ultrasonogram shows a hydatid cyst (1) in the right lobe of the liver (2). Daughter cysts (3) can be identified inside the large cyst. (Scanned 13cm above the umbilicus.)

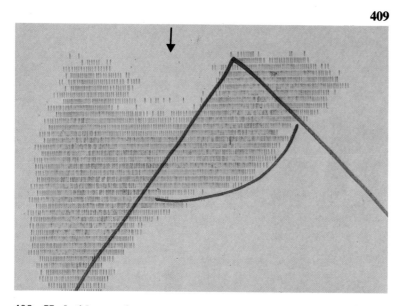

409. Hydatid cysts have caused the large filling defect (arrowed) in the liver in this [99]technetium isotope scan.

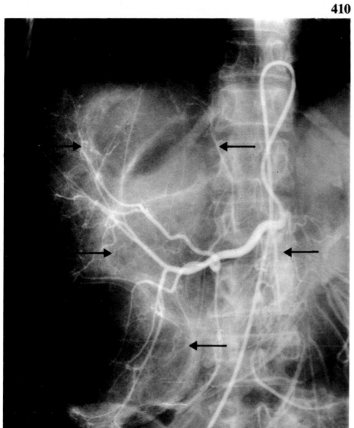

410. Hydatid cysts. A selective coeliac axis arteriogram may show stretching of vessels around the hydatid cysts. In this patient, the margins of three large cysts can be identified (arrowed).

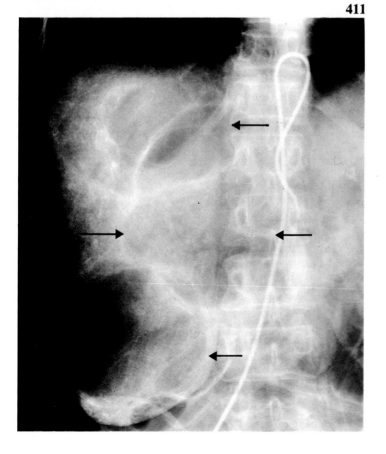

411. Hydatid cysts. In the venous phase of the coeliac axis arteriogram shown in **410** the cysts appear as avascular areas (arrowed).

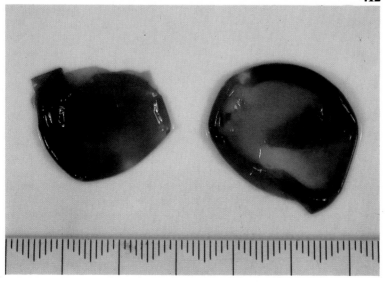

412. Hydatid cysts. These bile stained daughter cysts had obstructed the common bile duct. The patient presented with cholestatic jaundice due to rupture of a cyst into the biliary system.

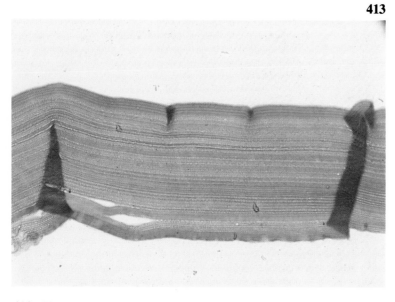

413. Hydatid cysts. Histological examination of a daughter cyst shown in **412** reveals the characteristic chitinous wall of a hydatid cyst. *(H. &E. ×63)*

Schistosomiasis (bilharziasis)

Schistosomiasis of the liver usually results from infestation with *S. mansoni* or *S. japonicum*. The infection is prevalent in Africa, the Far East and South America. Ova are excreted in the faeces and in water to become free swimming embryos. The embryos enter certain species of snails where they develop into cercariae. The cercariae leave the snails and gain access through the skin of bathers in infested water ('swimmer's itch'). The parasites migrate to the portal venous system where they develop into adult worms. The worms shed their eggs in the submucosal veins of the colon. Some of the eggs are carried in the portal venous blood back to the liver where they excite a hypersensitivity reaction with the formation of granulomas and fibrosis.

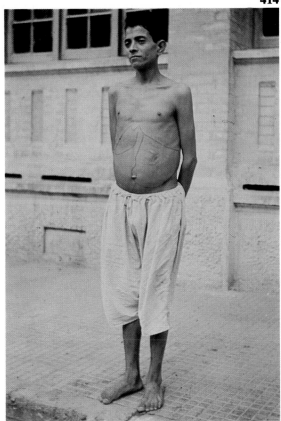

414. Schistosomiasis. The liver and spleen enlarge. Splenomegaly is due to portal hypertension. As the disease progresses, the liver shrinks and the spleen progressively enlarges. This Egyptian patient was infected with *S. mansoni*. He had a very large spleen and suffered repeated haematemeses from oesophageal varices.

415. Schistosomiasis. An enormous spleen may develop in this condition due to portal hypertension. In a selective coeliac axis arteriogram the splenic artery (1) has filled a huge spleen (2). The hepatic artery (3) is also filled. The patient presented with splenomegaly and haematemeses.

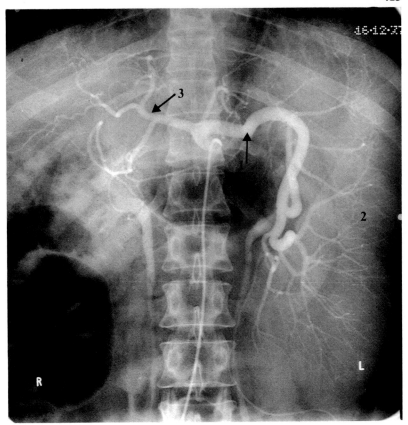

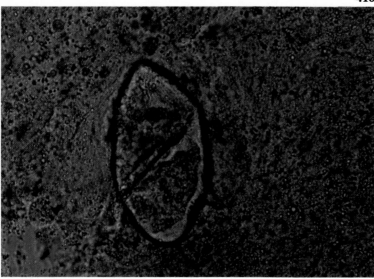

416. Schistosomiasis. A 'squash' preparation of part of a liver biopsy in glycerol may reveal the schistosomal eggs. This preparation showed a bluntly oval egg, measuring about $140 \times 60\mu$ with a lateral spine. This is the ovum of *S. mansoni.*

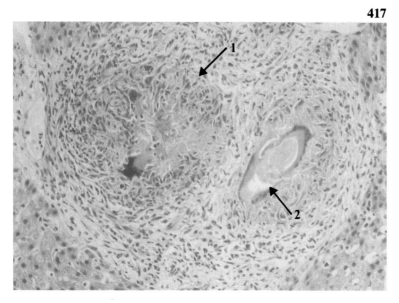

417. Schistosomiasis. The liver biopsy showed an enlarged portal tract containing a granuloma (1) and an ovum of *S. mansoni* (2). There is extensive fibrosis in the portal tract. Ova blocking the intrahepatic portal veins and the portal zone fibrosis lead to portal venous hypertension. *(H. & E. ×64)*

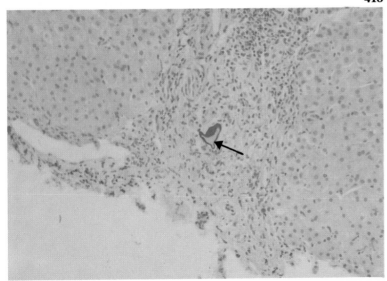

418. Schistosomiasis. The ova may be more readily identified by a Ziehl-Neelsen stain. In this liver biopsy the remnant of a schistosomal egg is stained deep pink in a fibrotic portal zone. *(×64)*

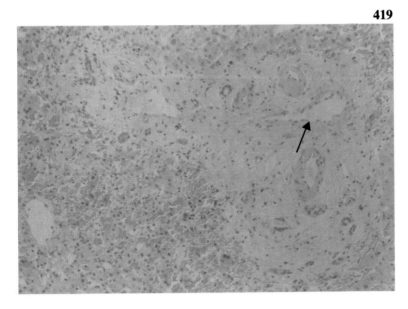

419. 'Pipe stem' fibrosis of the portal tracts may develop in schistosomiasis. This is associated with a heavy infestation of the adult worms. Dense fibrous septa extend from the granulomas. There is sclerosis around the walls of the portal veins (arrow). Bile duct proliferation and regenerative nodules are usually insignificant. *(H. & E. ×40)*

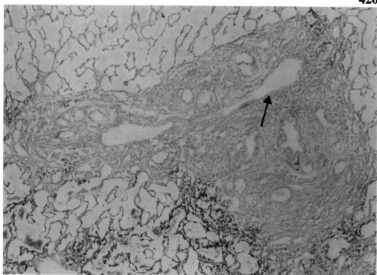

420. 'Pipe stem' fibrosis. A reticulin stain of the biopsy in **419** shows dense portal zone fibrosis containing the portal veins (arrowed). The surrounding reticulin architecture is preserved. *(×40)*

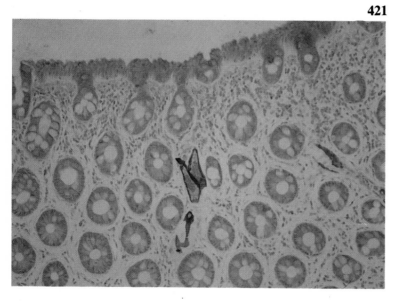

421. Schistosomiasis. Ova are often found in the rectum of patients with hepatic schistosomiasis. A Ziehl-Neelsen stain showed the dark pink staining walls of *S. mansoni* ova in this rectal biopsy. The patient's liver biopsy was shown in **416**.

Miscellaneous infections

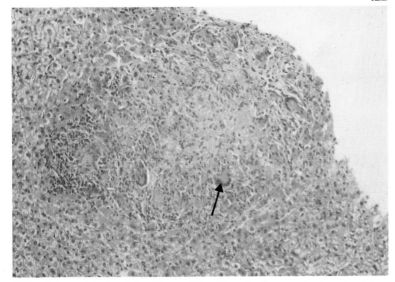

422. Tuberculosis of the liver. The liver is frequently involved in miliary tuberculosis. The commonest lesion is a caseating granuloma. This liver biopsy contains a large granuloma with lymphocytes, epithelioid cells and numerous giant cells (arrowed). The centre of the granuloma is caseating. Culture of the biopsy may yield tubercle bacilli. In some patients, extrahepatic signs of tuberculosis may not be obvious. *(H. & E. × 40)*

423

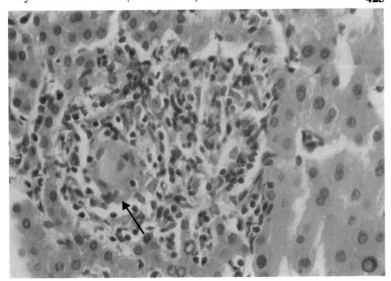

423. Sarcoidosis frequently involves the liver, causing widespread granuloma formation. The liver lesion is usually asymptomatic. An early sarcoid granuloma is a round, well-demarcated lesion commonly found in the portal tracts. The granuloma contains giant cells (arrowed) and pale staining epithelioid cells with a thin peripheral cuff of lymphocytes. In contrast to tuberculosis, there is no central caseation. *(H. & E. × 160)*

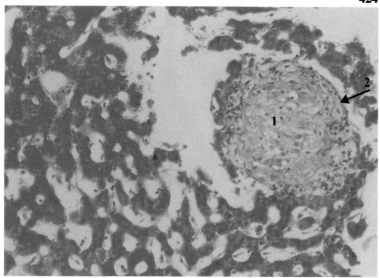

424. Sarcoidosis. Later in the course of the disease the granulomas develop a central area of acellular hyaline material (1) and a fibrous capsule. A peripheral ring of lymphocytes is present (2). The pallor of the granuloma is particularly marked in this biopsy stained for glycogen. *(Periodic acid Schiff×64)*

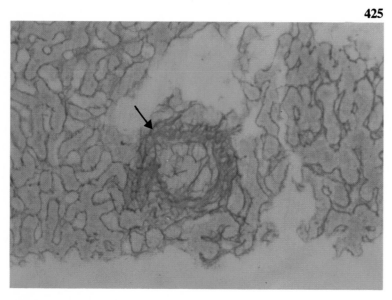

425. Sarcoidosis. A reticulin stain of the biopsy in **424** shows the fibrous capsule of a healing granuloma. The surrounding reticulin architecture is preserved. Portal hypertension is a rare late complication. *(×64)*

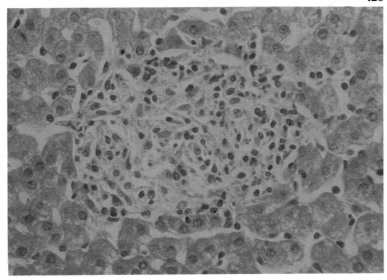

426. Brucellosis. Infection with *Brucella abortus* leads to widespread granuloma formation in the liver. The liver lesion is usually silent and hepatomegaly inconstant. The granulomas are indistinguishable from those of sarcoidosis. However, culture of part of the liver biopsy may yield the organism. In some patients, focal collections of lymphocytes, without granulomas are seen. *(H. & E. ×200)*

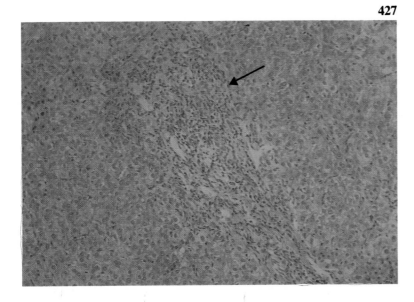

427. Syphilis. Occasionally hepatitis and jaundice complicate secondary syphilis. The clinical picture may simulate acute viral hepatitis. In some patients liver histology shows miliary granulomata. In others portal tract inflammation is the principal lesion. In this biopsy syphilis has resulted in portal zone infiltration (arrowed) with neutrophils and lymphocytes, foci of liver cell necrosis and cell 'drop-out'. The liver is also involved in congenital syphilis and in tertiary syphilis where gummas and a hepar lobatum may develop. *(H. & E. ×40)*

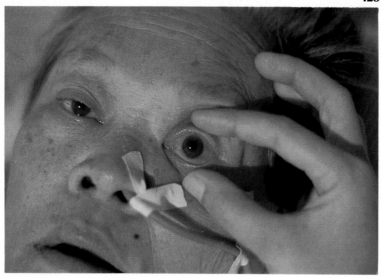

428. Leptospirosis. These infections are caused by a large group of leptospira including *L. icterohaemorrhagiae* (Weil's disease) and are usually spread by rats. The onset is abrupt with shivering followed by fever and marked prostration. Severe headaches, muscle and joint pains are common. Albuminuria is usual. This Thai patient shows the characteristic conjunctival suffusion of leptospirosis. There is great variation in the severity of the clinical course of these infections.

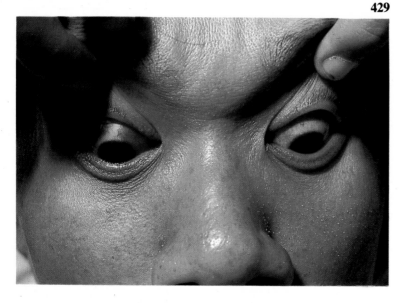

429. Leptospirosis. Jaundice appears between the 4th and 7th day in many patients and the liver is enlarged. The subconjunctival haemorrhage in this Thai patient is due to a bleeding tendency which usually accompanies severe attacks. Bleeding from the nose, gut and lungs, skin petechiae and ecchymoses may also develop.

430. Yellow fever is caused by a Group B arbovirus. An incubation period of three to six days is followed by headache, backache and prostration. Hypotension, jaundice, albuminuria, widespread haemorrhages and vomiting of altered blood may develop. A liver biopsy shows severe liver cell necrosis particularly in the mid-zonal areas (arrowed) and Councilman bodies. Inflammatory cells are characteristically scanty. *(H. & E. ×8)*

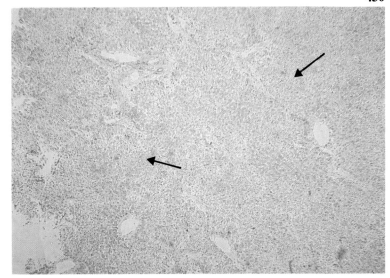

430a. Lassa fever is a viral disease encountered in West Africa which causes a 'haemorrhagic fever'. The patients develop headache, fever, muscle pains and pharyngitis. Vomiting, diarrhoea, proteinuria and a bleeding tendency may develop later. A liver biopsy shows widespread eosinophilic necrosis of liver cells without inflammatory cells. The liver changes may appear similar to yellow fever, except that in Lassa fever, necrosis develops in all areas of the lobule. *(H. & E. ×8)*

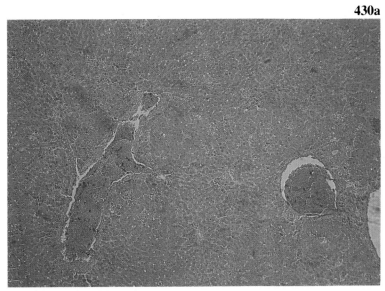

431. Infectious mononucleosis may involve the liver and mimic infectious hepatitis. A liver biopsy shows the portal tracts (arrowed) and sinusoids infiltrated with large mononuclear cells. Focal areas of liver cell necrosis develop but unlike infective hepatitis centrizonal necrosis is not present. *(H. & E. ×64)*

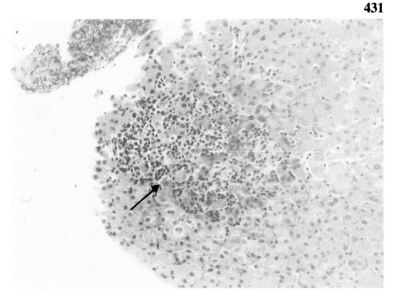

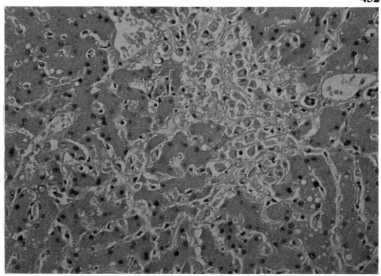

432. Marburg virus hepatitis has been contracted by laboratory workers from the Vervet (African Green Monkey). The incubation period is between four and seven days. Headache, pyrexia, vomiting, central nervous system involvement and a hepatitis develop. This rare disease is severe and a proportion of the patients have died. A liver biopsy shows areas of centrizonal necrosis containing numerous acidophilic bodies. Fatty change may also develop. *(H. & E. ×64)*

433

434

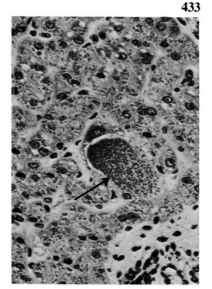

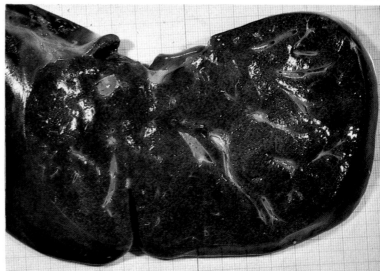

433. Malaria. The liver is infected during the pre-erythrocytic stage. Sporozoites from a mosquito invade liver cells where they divide to form a 'tissue' schizont (arrowed). The liver cell enlarges and finally ruptures liberating many merozoites which enter erythrocytes (erythrocytic stage). There are usually no specific signs of liver involvement in malaria. *(Giemsa-colophonium×350)*

434. Malaria. In chronic infections a brown pigment accumulates in the liver and spleen. This section of liver shows the typical dark brown appearance of chronic malaria. It is due to iron and haemofucsin in the Kupffer cells.

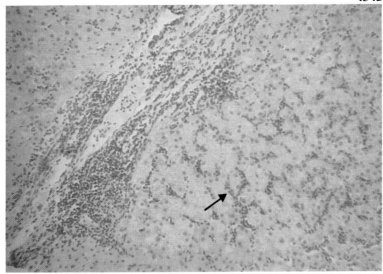

434a. Tropical splenomegaly syndrome. An abnormal immune response to malarial infection may result in marked splenomegaly. The serum IgM concentration is always elevated. A liver biopsy shows dilated sinusoids (arrowed) heavily infiltrated with lymphocytes and hypertrophied Kupffer cells. *(H. & E. × 40)*

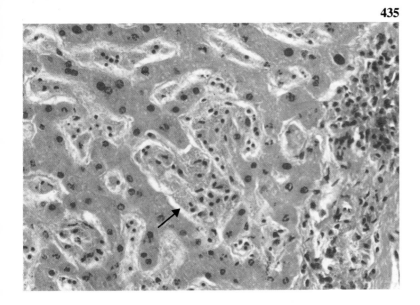

435. Kala-azar (leishmaniasis) is a protozoan infection involving the reticulo-endothelial system causing fevers and marked hepatosplenomegaly. A liver biopsy shows enlarged Kupffer cells (arrowed) distending the sinusoids. The Kupffer cells contain Leishman-Donovan bodies. The portal tracts are infiltrated with chronic inflammatory cells. *(H. & E. × 100)*

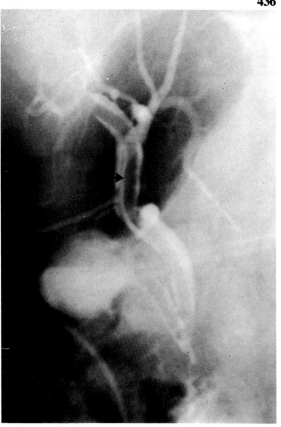

436. Ascariasis. The round worm *Ascaris lumbricoides* may lodge in the common bile duct causing partial biliary obstruction and cholangitis with liver abscesses. Haemobilia is a further complication. Biliary ascariasis is usually encountered in the Far East. This operative cholangiogram shows a large round worm (arrowed) in a dilated common bile duct. The worm usually dies in the bile duct and may calcify.

437

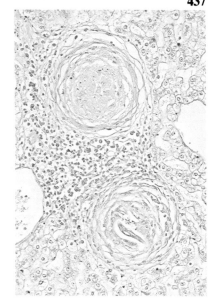

437. Toxocariasis. This worm, which is spread by dogs *(Toxocara canis)* and cats *(T. cati)*, invades many tissues (visceral larva migrans). Infestation of the liver results in granuloma formation. The signs of liver involvement are non-specific. A marked blood eosinophilia is usual. *(×150)*

Liver flukes

438

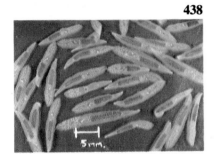

438. Clonorchis sinensis. The Chinese liver fluke is found in Eastern Asia. The mature fluke may reach 2cm in length. Man is infected by eating raw or partly cooked fish. The migration of the flukes to the biliary tree is usually accompanied by a pyrexia and a blood eosinophilia.

438a

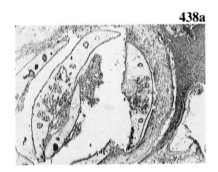

438a. Clonorchis sinensis. This liver section shows the flukes in a bile duct where they cause severe fibrosis and adenomatous change *(×15)*. Bile duct obstruction, caused by these flukes, is frequently complicated by bacterial cholangitis, multiple liver abscesses and intrahepatic gallstone formation. *Bile duct carcinoma* and *primary liver cancer* may develop later.

439

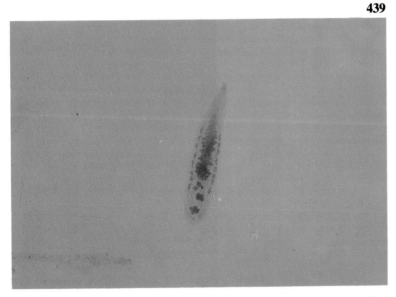

439. Opisthorchis viverrini. These liver flukes are found in Northeast Thailand, Laos and Cambodia. Uncooked fish is the usual source of infestation. *O. viverrini* causes similar biliary disease to *C. sinensis*.

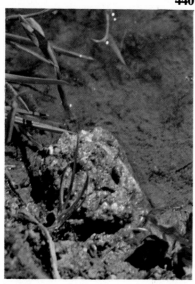

440. Ecology of fasciola hepatica. Sheep and cattle are usually infected. The intermediate hosts, Lymnaea snails, thrive in wet pasture and excrete the encysted cercariae of the flukes. Man is usually infected by eating wild watercress. This picture shows the common British intermediate host, *L. trunculata*, in a typical wet habitat.

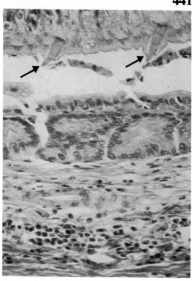

441. Fasciola hepatica invade the biliary system causing cholangitis with fever, pain and hepatomegaly. A blood eosinophilia usually develops. The clinical picture may simulate gallstones in the common bile duct. The spines of the fluke (arrowed) damage the biliary epithelium. *(×350)*

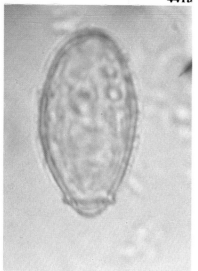

441a. Liver flukes. The diagnosis can be confirmed by finding ova in the faeces. This is the ovum of *O. viverrini. (×500)*

9. Fibropolycystic disease of the liver and biliary system

Fibropolycystic disease encompasses a large group of rare congenital hepato-biliary diseases. These include adult fibropolycystic disease (polycystic liver), congenital hepatic fibrosis, congenital intrahepatic biliary dilatation (Caroli's disease) and choledochal cysts. Associated kidney defects are common. Malignant change may complicate congenital hepatic fibrosis, Caroli's disease and choledochal cysts.

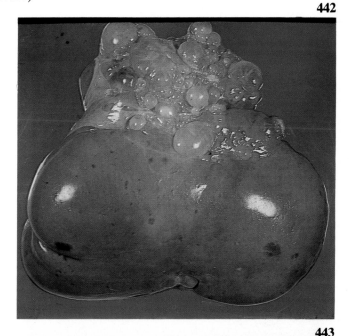

442

442. Adult fibropolycystic disease. The liver contains many thin walled cysts filled with a clear or brown-coloured fluid due to altered blood. The cysts vary in size from a pinhead to about 10cm in diameter. The remainder of the liver is normal. In many cases a polycystic liver is an incidental finding at autopsy. Occasionally, patients present with a nodular swelling in the upper abdomen due to enlarging cysts.

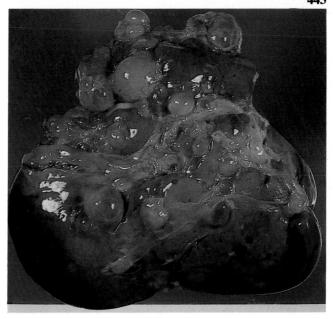

443

443. Adult fibropolycystic disease. The inferior surface of the liver in **442** contains many more cysts of varying sizes.

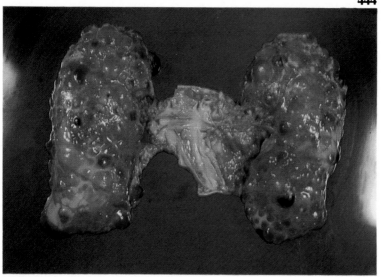

444. Adult fibropolycystic disease. Polycystic kidneys were present in the patient shown in **442**. Patients with adult fibropolycystic disease may present with renal complications including renal failure.

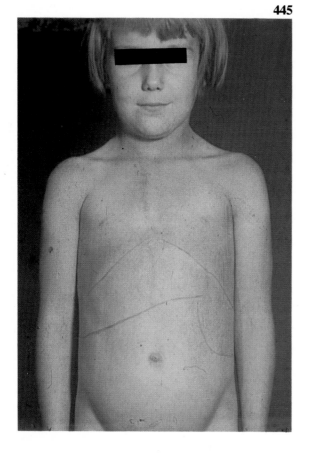

445. Congenital hepatic fibrosis. This rare condition is usually diagnosed before 10 years of age. Children present with a large, very hard liver, splenomegaly or bleeding from oesophageal varices. Note the hepato-splenomegaly in this child. The vein on the abdominal wall is a portal systemic collateral caused by portal venous hypertension. Her development was normal. Congenital hepatic fibrosis may be misdiagnosed as cirrhosis. Abnormalities of the biliary system, such as Caroli's disease or choledochal cysts may also be present.

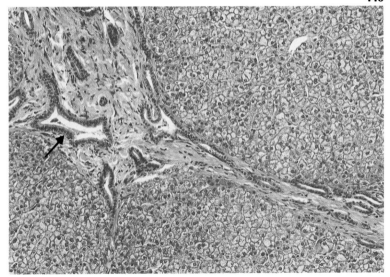

446. Congenital hepatic fibrosis. A liver biopsy reveals normal hepatic lobules encased by broad collagenous fibrous bands. Well developed bile ducts (arrowed) are present in the fibrous bands. *(H. & E. ×40)*

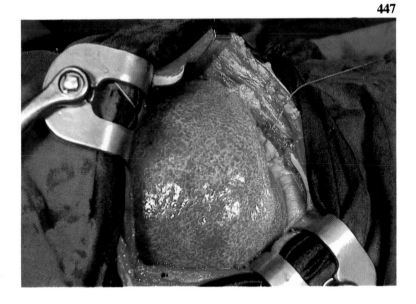

447. Congenital hepatic fibrosis. The liver feels hard and the surface has a mottled white appearance due to the thick fibrous bands. The tough texture of the liver may make a percutaneous liver biopsy difficult.

448. Congenital hepatic fibrosis. A splenic venogram shows a large leash of oesophageal varices (1) arising from the left gastric vein (2) in this child. Portal venous hypertension has caused retrograde flow down the inferior mesenteric vein (3). The intrahepatic portal veins (4) have been distorted and pruned by the hepatic fibrosis.

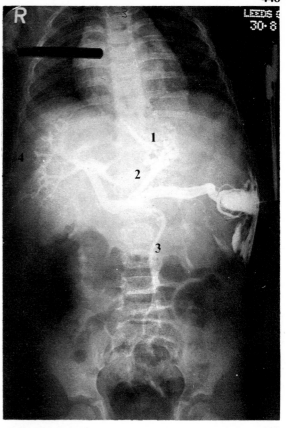

449. Medullary sponge kidney is the usual renal disease associated with congenital hepatic fibrosis. Spotty areas of calcification (arrowed) develop in a medullary sponge kidney. These are small cysts adjacent to the renal calyces.

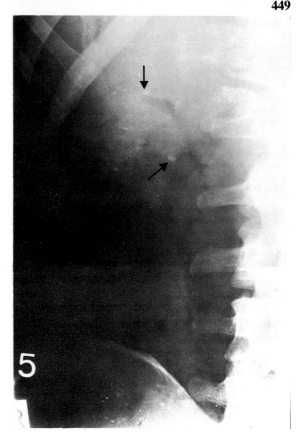

450. Congenital intrahepatic biliary dilatation (Caroli's disease). An endoscopic retrograde cholangiogram shows saccular dilatations (arrowed) of the intrahepatic bile ducts. The rest of the biliary tree is normal. The patients usually present in childhood or early adulthood with episodes of abdominal pain, cholangitis and Gram-negative septicaemia. Stones may develop in the dilated intrahepatic bile ducts. This patient also had congenital hepatic fibrosis.

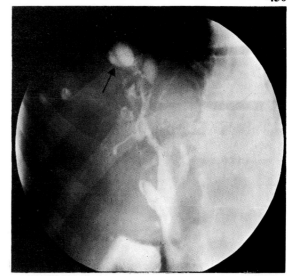

451. Choledochal cyst is a congenital dilatation of a part or whole of the common bile duct. It is more common in girls and usually appears in childhood. Choledochal cysts classically cause a triad of intermittent pain, jaundice and a right hypochondrial mass. This 20-year-old girl presented with recurrent acute pancreatitis due to stones in the cyst obstructing the pancreatic duct. She was never jaundiced. The endoscopic retrograde cholangiogram showed a massively dilated common bile duct. The gall bladder was normal, but obscured by the dilated bile duct.

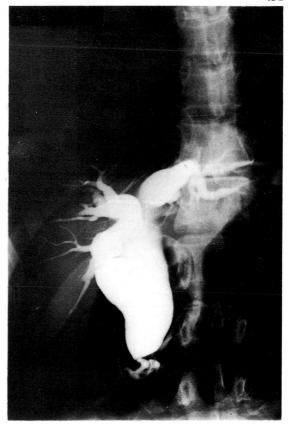

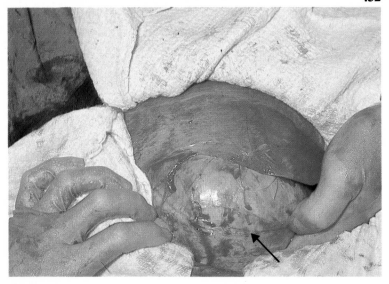

452. Solitary liver cyst. These are rare, presenting with abdominal distension, hepatomegaly or pressure effects on adjacent organs. They usually develop on the antero-inferior surface of the liver as in this patient with a very large cyst weighing 4.5kg (arrowed). The cyst is multiloculated and contains a clear or brown-coloured fluid.

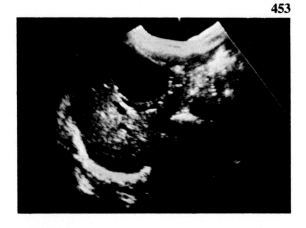 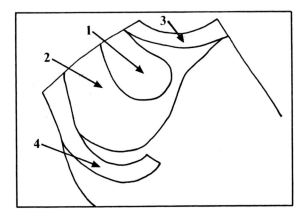

453. Solitary liver cyst. This patient presented with hepatomegaly. Grey scale ultrasonography showed a solitary cyst (1) in the right lobe of the liver (2) under the anterior abdominal wall (3). The diaphragm is also shown (4). (Scanned 14cm above the umbilicus.)

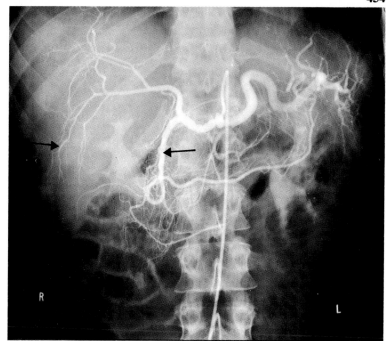

454. Solitary liver cyst. A selective coeliac axis arteriogram showed displacement and stretching of the intrahepatic vessels (arrowed) by the cyst shown in **453**.

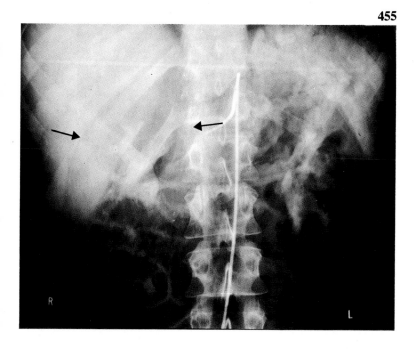

455. Solitary liver cyst. In the venous phase of the coeliac axis arteriogram, the cyst appears as an avascular filling defect (arrowed).

10. Tumours of the liver and biliary system

Primary hepato-cellular carcinoma

The incidence of primary liver cancer shows wide geographical variations. It is a common cancer in Africa and South East Asia but rare in temperate climates. Predisposing factors include cirrhosis, type B viral hepatitis, haemochromatosis and androgenic steroids, such as methyltestosterone and oxymethalone. Food carcinogens, such as aflatoxin, may be important in some areas.

456. Primary liver cancer. This patient, with alcoholic cirrhosis, had stopped taking alcohol several years before. He presented with abdominal pain due to a rapidly enlarging liver. A primary liver cancer was present in the right lobe. Note the scanty body hair and muscle wasting. **456**

457. Primary liver cancer may cause sudden clinical deterioration in a cirrhotic patient. The appearance of ascites in this woman with well compensated inactive cirrhosis heralded the diagnosis of a primary liver cancer. Note the scanty body hair, everted umbilicus and abdominal wall veins. **457**

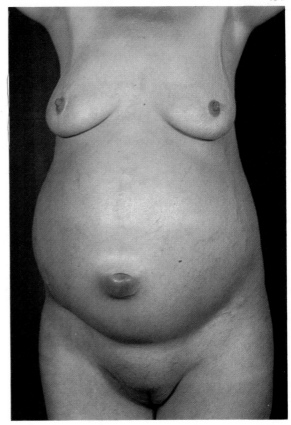

458. Primary liver cancer in a 40-year-old Arab woman presented as a mass in the right hypochondrium (arrowed). She had chronic type B viral hepatitis. An arterial bruit could be heard over the mass.

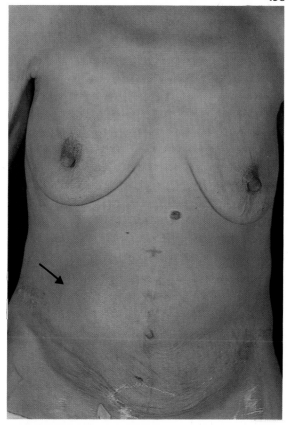

459. Abdominal x-ray of the patient in **458** showed a huge liver with a large round mass in the right lobe (arrowed).

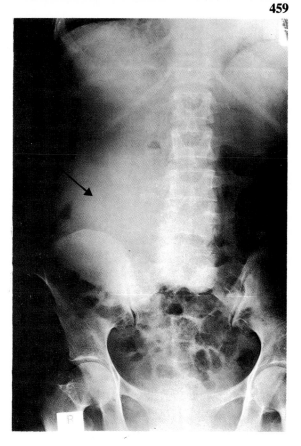

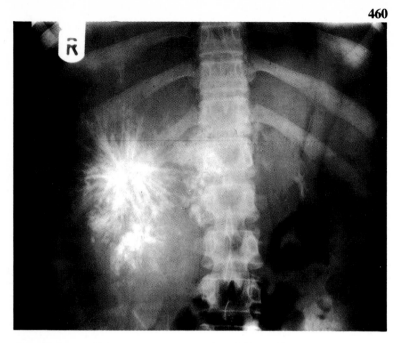

460. Primary liver cancer may rarely calcify. This abdominal x-ray shows 'sun burst' calcification in a primary liver cancer.

461

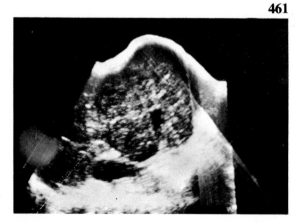 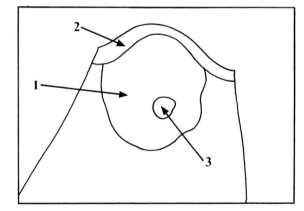

461. Grey scale ultrasonography of the patient in **458** showed a large round primary liver cancer (1) pushing out the anterior abdominal wall (2). The cavity (3) in the centre of the tumour is due to necrosis. (Sagittal scan 6.5cm right of the umbilicus).

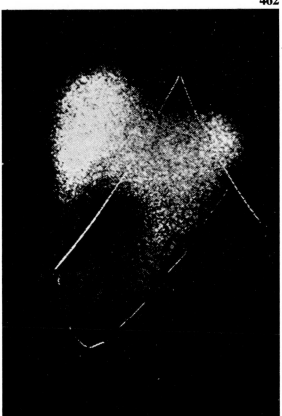

462. Isotope scan. A tumour in the right lobe of the liver caused a large filling defect in this ^{99}technetium scan.

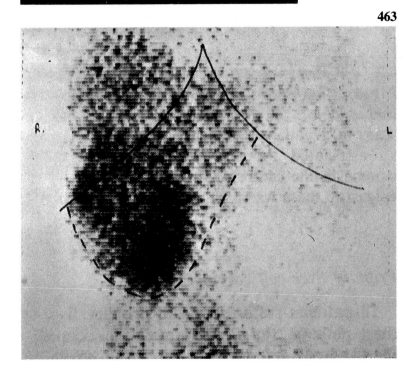

463. Isotope scan. ^{67}Gallium citrate was taken up by the tumour shown in **462**, confirming that it was a primary liver cancer.

464. Coeliac axis arteriography is valuable in the diagnosis of these vascular cancers. The intrahepatic arteries are displaced and stretched (1) around the tumour. The vessels inside the tumour are irregular and fragmented (2). In contrast, secondary malignant deposits in the liver tend to be avascular. This is the arteriogram of the patient in **458**.

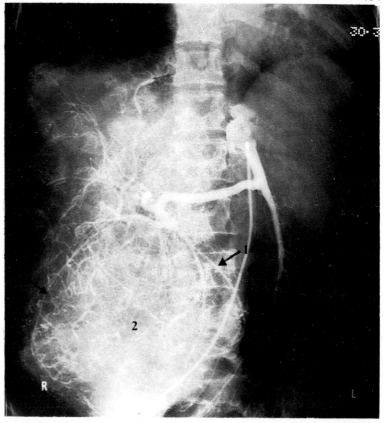

465. Primary liver cancer metastases caused the round shadows in the lungs of this six-year-old girl. Other sites for metastases are the supraclavicular fossae, bones and brain. The enlarged liver has elevated the right hemidiaphragm.

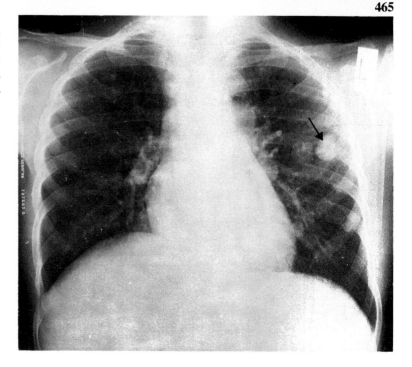

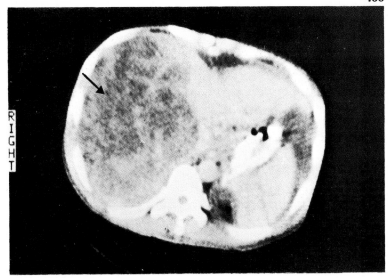

466. Computerised tomography in a 36-year-old Chinese man shows a large, moderately vascular primary liver cancer (arrowed) in the right lobe of the liver. The portal vein was blocked. He presented with abdominal pain, swelling and haematemeses. Hepatomegaly and oesophageal varices were present and a test for HBsAg was positive.

467

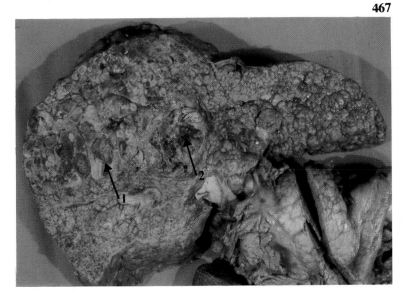

467. Primary liver cancer was confirmed at the autopsy of the patient in **466**. The cirrhotic liver contained a large tumour (1) in the right lobe. The portal vein was thrombosed (2).

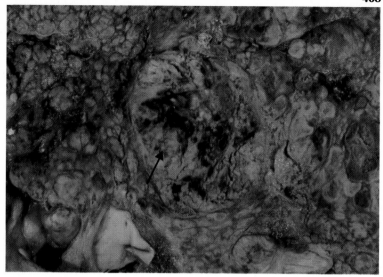

468. Primary liver cancer. A close-up view of the liver in **467** shows thrombus occluding the portal vein (arrowed). The surrounding liver is studded with pale nodules of primary liver cancer. Some of the nodules are haemorrhagic and necrotic. Portal vein thrombosis followed invasion of the portal vein by the tumour.

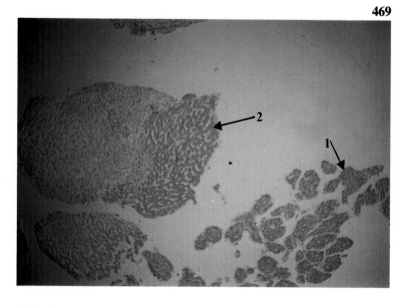

469. Liver biopsy in this patient yielded fragments of primary liver cancer (1) and nodules of cirrhotic liver (2). Fragmented biopsies are commonly encountered in cirrhotic patients. *(Best's carmine×50)*

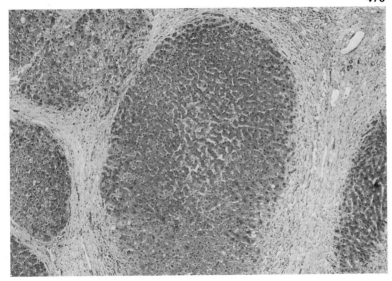

470. Primary liver cancer usually develops in an inactive cirrhosis. In another part of this cirrhotic liver, the tumour illustrated in **471** was found. *(H. & E. ×40)*

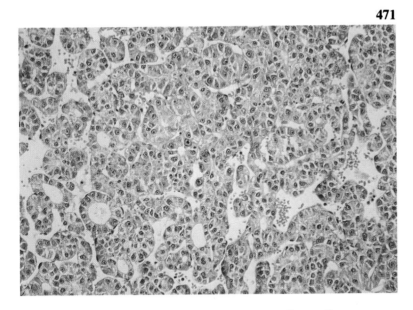

471. Primary liver cancer cells resemble normal liver cells to a varying extent depending on the differentiation of the tumour. A higher magnification shows the tumour cells to be smaller than normal with large hyperchromatic nuclei. Mitoses are prominent. Some of the cells form pseudo-tubules. Between the cells are large blood filled spaces but little intercellular stroma. *(H. & E. ×64)*

Adenomas of the liver

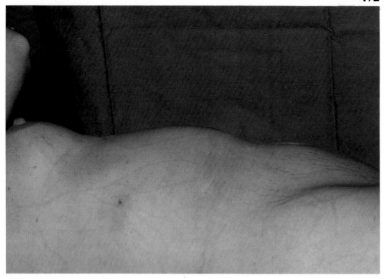

472. Liver adenomas are very rare tumours. In some patients there appears to be an association with oral contraceptive drugs. This 33-year-old American woman had taken oral contraceptives for five years when she developed pain and swelling in the right hypochondrium. Liver adenomas may rupture causing massive intraperitoneal haemorrhage.

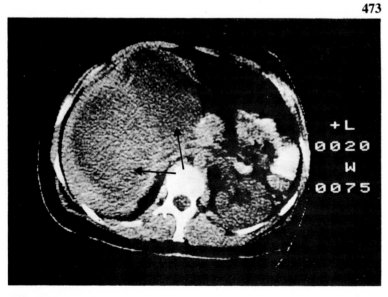

473. Computerised tomography of the abdomen of the patient in **472** showed a large lobulated tumour (arrowed) in the right lobe of the liver.

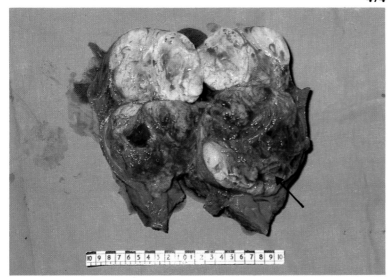

474. Liver adenoma removed surgically from the patient in **472**. Note the white lobulated tumour. Haemorrhage into one of the nodules (arrowed) has formed a blood filled cavity.

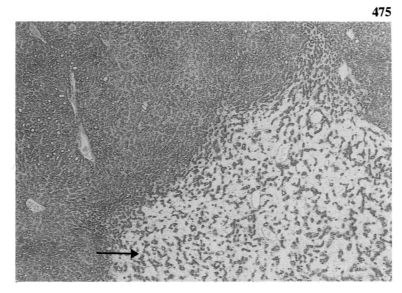

475. Liver adenomas. The liver cells and bile ducts appear normal but are not organised to form lobules. Note the necrotic centre (arrowed) of this tumour. *(H. & E. ×10)*

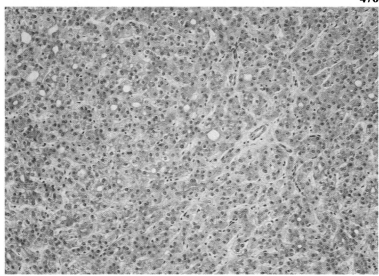

476. Liver adenoma. A higher magnification shows the normal liver cells but no normal liver lobules, i.e. absence of portal tracts. *(H. & E. × 40)*

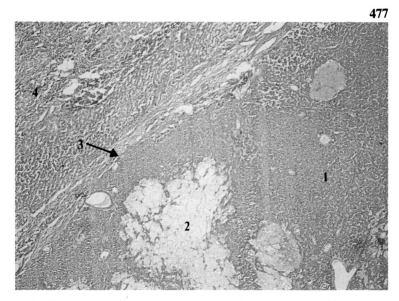

477. Peliosis hepatis may develop in a liver adenoma (1) causing large blood-filled spaces (2). A fibrous capsule (3) surrounds the adenoma separating it from the normal liver (4). This adenoma was associated with the oral contraceptive pill. *(H. & E. × 10)*

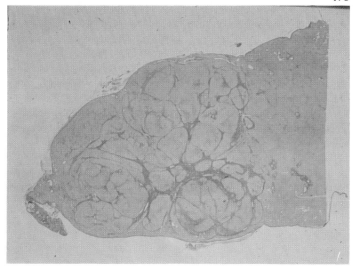

478. Focal nodular hyperplasia are firm solitary areas of liver usually found in women. They are commonly subcapsular. Fibrous septa radiate from a central core. Focal nodular hyperplasia must be distinguished from a liver adenoma. *(Picro-Mallory)*

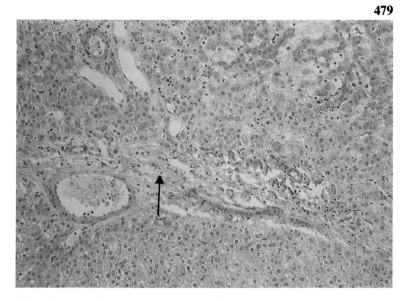

479. Focal nodular hyperplasia. A liver biopsy shows an encapsulated area of nodular hyperplasia containing prominent hyperplastic blood vessels and bile ducts. A focal stellate scar is arrowed. *(H. & E. × 40)*

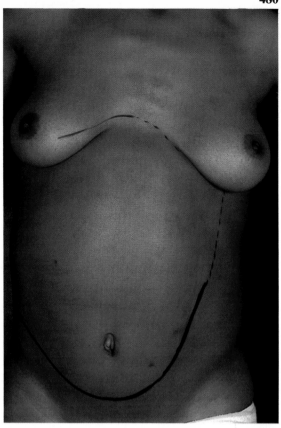

480. Cystadenomas of the liver are very rare tumours, derived either from bile duct cells (cholangioma) or both bile duct and hepatic cells (mixed tumours). Cystadenomas are multiloculated and may grow very large as in this patient. They must be distinguished from fibropolycystic disease and solitary cysts of the liver.

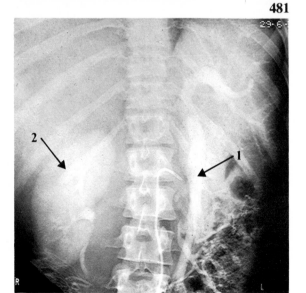

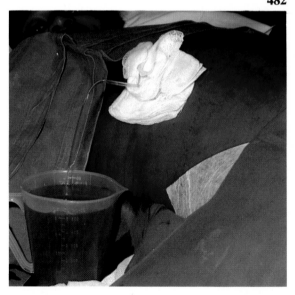

481. Cystadenoma of the liver. The venous phase of a coeliac axis arteriogram from the patient in **480** showed a large liver tumour displacing the portal vein (1) to a bizarre position. A normal right kidney (2) is opacified behind the tumour.

482. Cystadenoma of the liver. A percutaneous catheter introduced into the cyst drained a greeny-brown fluid.

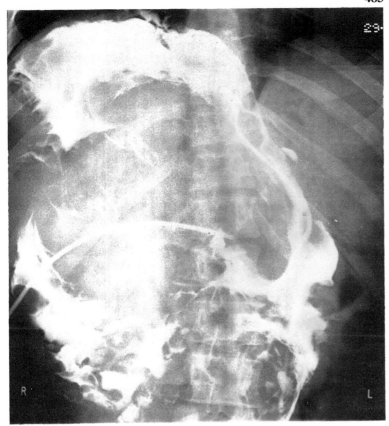

483. Cystadenoma of the liver. Contrast medium injected through the catheter shows the extent of this multiloculated cystic tumour.

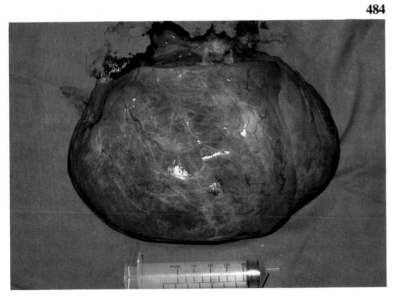

484. Cystadenoma of the liver. After drainage of the cyst, a large tumour was removed from the patient in **480**.

Tumours of blood vessels in the liver

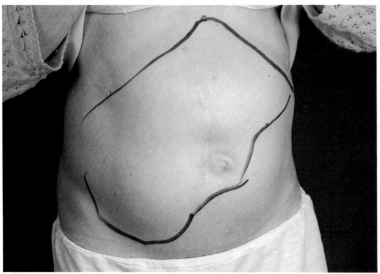

485. Haemangiomas are rare and often incidental findings at autopsy. Occasionally, as in this patient, they are the cause of hepatomegaly. A vascular hum may be heard over the liver. Spontaneous rupture can occur.

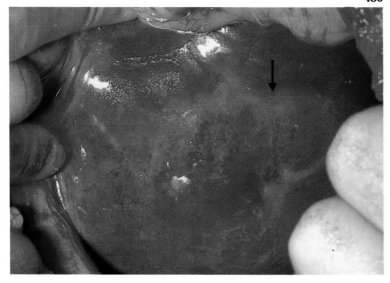

486. Haemangioma of the liver usually appears as a dark red subcapsular tumour on the convexity of the right lobe.

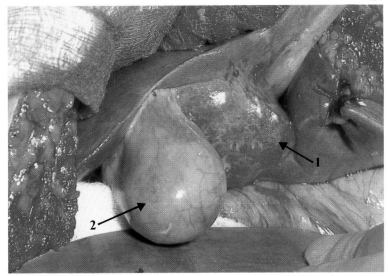

487. Haemangioma. On the inferior surface of the liver shown in **486** a pedunculated haemangioma (1) had developed adjacent to the gall bladder (2).

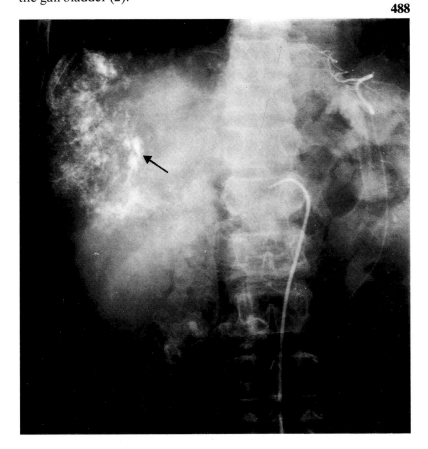

488. Haemangiomas in the liver are well demonstrated by selective coeliac axis arteriography. The vascular spaces of the haemangioma (arrowed) fill with contrast and remain opacified for a prolonged period after the injection.

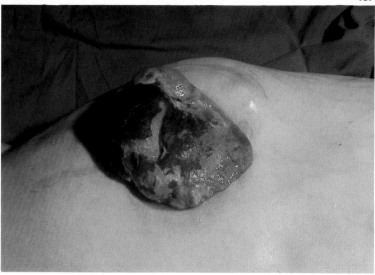

489. Haemangiosarcoma is a very rare and highly malignant tumour usually developing in childhood. The liver rapidly enlarges with nodular, cavernous growths. Blood stained ascites usually develops. A vascular bruit may be heard over the liver. In this patient the dark vascular tumour had penetrated through the anterior abdominal wall. Exposure to *thorotrast* and *vinyl chloride monomers* have been associated with the development of haemangiosarcoma.

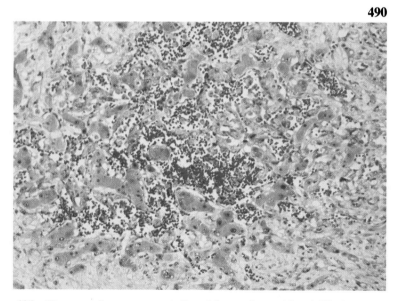

490. Haemangiosarcoma. A liver biopsy shows blood filled spaces lined by layers of highly malignant anaplastic endothelial cells. *(H. & E. ×40)*

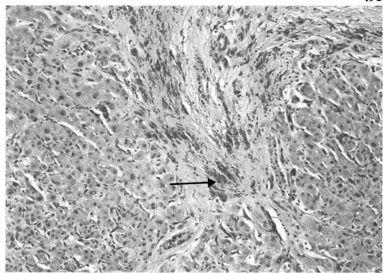

491. Thorotrast, a colloidal solution of the radioactive isotope thorium dioxide, was formerly used as a contrast agent in radiology. Thorotrast (arrowed) accumulates in the liver. Years later malignant tumours may develop including primary liver cancer, bile duct cancer and haemangiosarcoma. Thorotrast may also cause cirrhosis.

Secondary tumours of the liver

The liver is the commonest site for metastases from malignant tumours. Metastases usually spread to the liver via the blood. Deposits from cancer of the lung, breast, colon, stomach and pancreas are most frequently encountered.

492. Secondary cancer of the liver usually presents with an enlarged very hard liver. This patient had metastases from carcinoma of stomach. The liver may become enormous, reaching the iliac crest. The liver surface often feels irregular. Patients frequently complain of fullness and swelling in the abdomen and a dragging sensation. General clinical deterioration and muscle wasting are usually rapid.

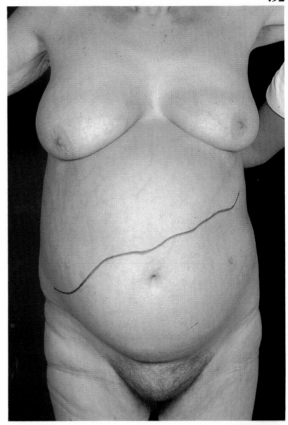

493. Secondary cancer. Metastatic deposits should be sought in other sites. In this patient, with carcinoma of the stomach, metastases (arrowed) were present in the lymph nodes of the left supraclavicular fossa (Virchow's node).

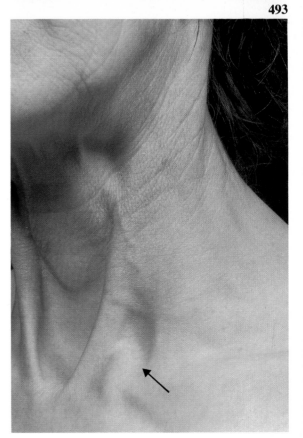

493

494. Secondary cancer. A metastasis from cancer of the pancreas in the umbilicus of this patient caused the painless, purple swelling.

494

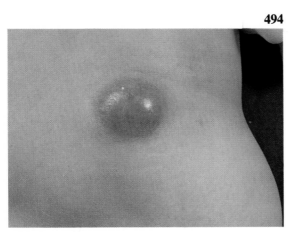

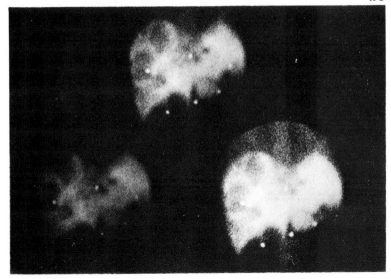

495. Secondary cancer. A [99]technetium isotope scan shows multiple filling defects in the liver. The primary tumour was cancer of the colon.

496

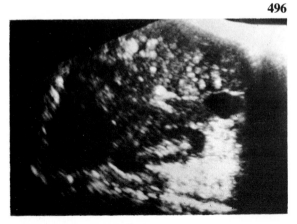 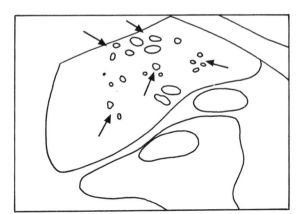

496. Secondary cancer. Grey scale ultrasonography demonstrated multiple nodules (arrowed) in the liver of this patient. These were metastases from cancer of the pancreas.

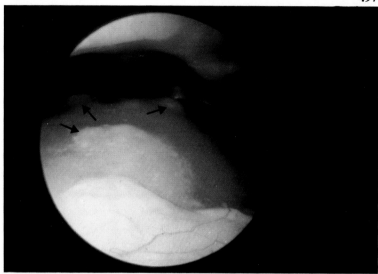

497. Secondary cancer. Peritoneoscopy in this patient showed the liver surface studded with metastases (arrowed). The primary tumour was cancer of the pancreas. This technique permits direct biopsy of the nodules.

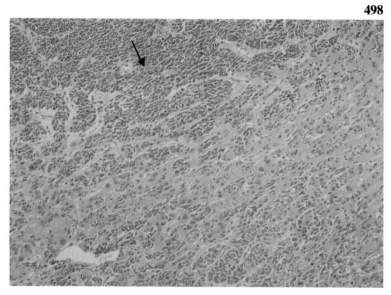

498. Secondary cancer. A percutaneous liver biopsy often reveals metastases in the liver. This patient presented with hepatomegaly. The liver biopsy showed a metastasis from a bronchial carcinoma (arrowed). Sheets of small dark malignant cells are invading the pale pink liver tissue. The primary tumour was not visible on a chest x-ray. *(H. & E. ×40)*

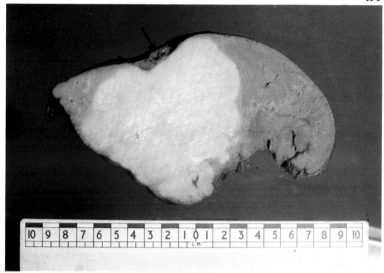

499. Secondary cancer. A large pale metastasis from adeno-carcinoma of the colon is present in this section of the liver. The surface of the liver is umbilicated (arrowed). This is due to necrosis and subsequent shrinkage of the metastasis.

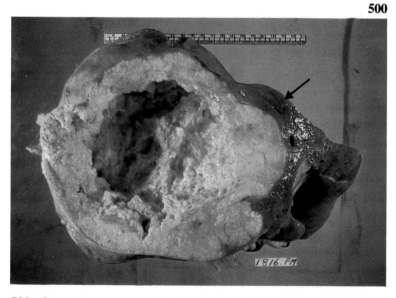

500. Secondary cancer. Central necrosis of a liver metastasis may lead to the formation of a cavity. This results when the enlarging tumour outgrows its blood supply. The primary tumour was a squamous carcinoma of the bronchus. A thin lining of normal liver can be seen (arrowed).

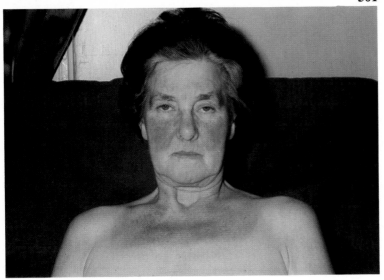

501. Carcinoid syndrome. Liver metastases from a gastro-intestinal carcinoid tumour caused flushing attacks in this woman. Note the violaceous colour of her cheeks. The remainder of her face and the necklace area are also flushed. Diarrhoea and valvular lesions of the heart may develop. The primary tumour is usually found in the appendix, ileum or jejunum. Symptoms only develop when liver metastases are present.

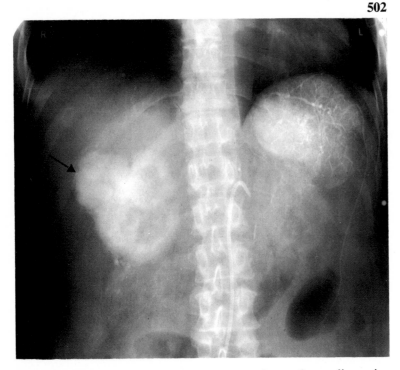

502. Carcinoid syndrome. In the venous phase of a coeliac axis arteriogram from the patient in **501** the circular blushes (arrowed) are carcinoid metastases. Endocrine tumour metastases typically cause marked venous blushing.

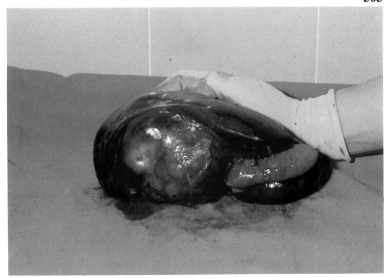

503. Carcinoid tumour metastases are the pale deposits in the liver of the patient shown in **501**.

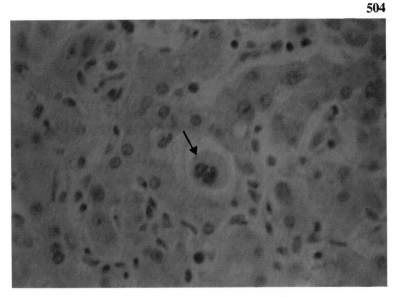

504. Myeloid metaplasia in the liver may follow irritation or replacement of the bone marrow by secondary carcinoma. It also develops in myelosclerosis, multiple myeloma and marble bone disease (Albers-Schönberg disease). A leuco-erythroblastic anaemia is commonly present. Liver biopsy shows increased cellularity in the sinusoids and portal tracts. These contain a variety of cells at different stages of maturation including giant cells (arrowed) which resemble megakaryocytes. *(H. & E. ×175)*

Tumours affecting the biliary system

505. Carcinoma of the intrahepatic bile ducts usually affects older people and causes a cholestatic (obstructive type) jaundice. The level of icterus may fluctuate but eventually the patient becomes deeply jaundiced. Hepatomegaly is usual but the extra-hepatic biliary tree and gall bladder are collapsed. The serum bilirubin level in this patient was 35mg/100ml (595μmol/l).

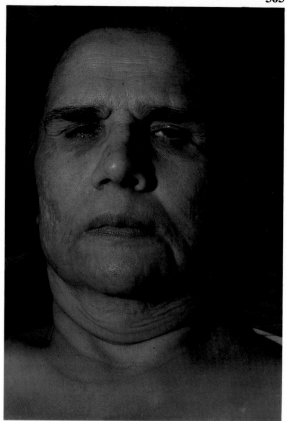

506. Intrahepatic bile duct cancer is usually slow growing and patients may survive for years. This patient had been jaundiced for five years. The xanthelasmas around her eyes are the result of prolonged cholestasis.

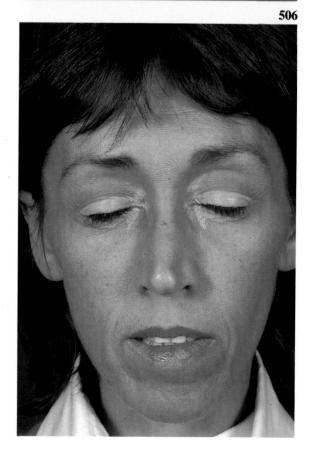

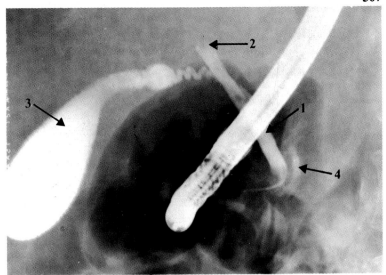

507. Intrahepatic bile duct cancer. An endoscopic retrograde cholangiogram may only fill the biliary system below the stricture. The common bile duct (1) is of normal calibre and terminates bluntly at the porta hepatis (2). The gall bladder (3) is not dilated. The pancreatic duct (4) has also been filled.

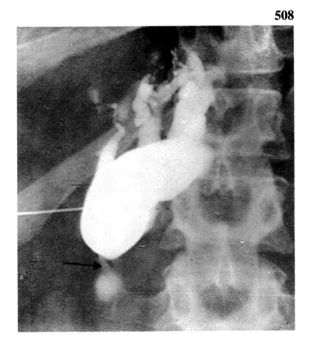

508. Intrahepatic bile duct cancer. A percutaneous cholangiogram from the patient in **507** shows a grossly dilated intrahepatic biliary tree above the malignant stricture (arrow).

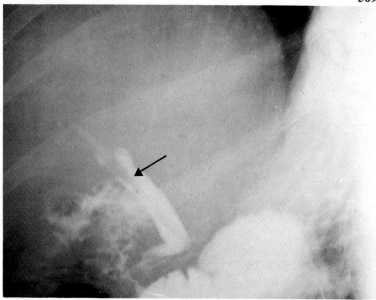

509. Intrahepatic bile duct cancer. Surgical removal is usually not possible. A plastic tube pushed through the tumour may provide adequate drainage and relief of the jaundice. In this patient, jaundice reappeared 18 months after the insertion of a plastic tube (arrowed). Tumour and debris prevented the entry of the contrast medium into the tube in this endoscopic retrograde cholangiogram.

510

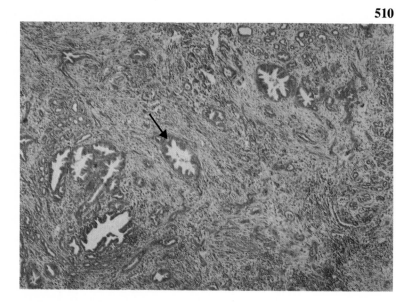

510. Intrahepatic bile duct cancers are usually firm, fibrous tumours. The malignant cells are arranged into tubules resembling bile ducts (arrowed) and are surrounded by dense fibrous tissue. Histologically, the tumours are scirrhous, mucus-secreting adenocarcinomas. *(H. & E. ×13)*

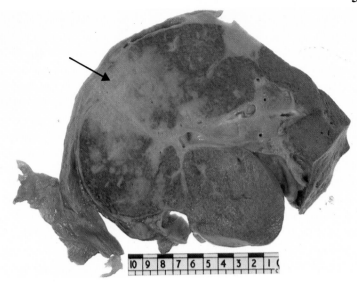

511. Intrahepatic bile duct cancer (arrowed) has spread along the bile ducts and into the liver parenchyma. This patient had survived for seven years. Note the dark green, nodular liver. Secondary biliary cirrhosis had developed.

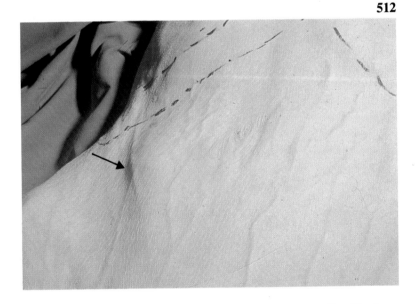

512. Cancer of the pancreas is a common tumour usually affecting the middle aged and elderly. Cancer of the head of the pancreas may obstruct the lower end of the common bile duct. A cholestatic (obstructive type) jaundice results. Prominent symptoms are jaundice, weight loss and dull abdominal pain. Hepatomegaly is usual. The extrahepatic biliary tree is dilated and in some patients the gall bladder (arrowed) is palpable or even visible (Courvoisier's law).

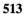

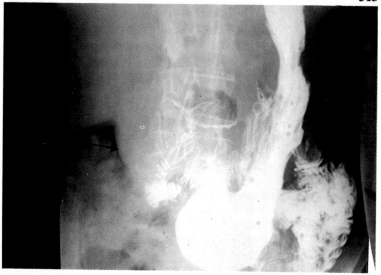

513. Cancer of the pancreas. An x-ray of the abdomen may reveal an enlarged gall bladder (arrowed) compressing the duodenum.

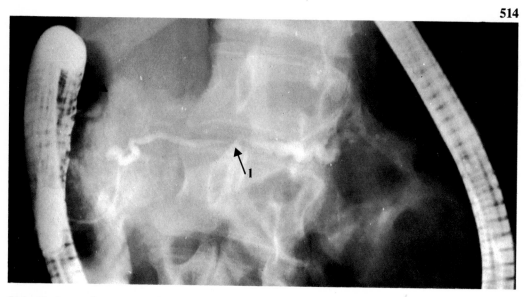

514. Endoscopic retrograde pancreatography in a patient with cancer of the pancreas shows a malignant stricture (1) in the mid-portion of the pancreatic duct. The duct distal to the stricture is dilated. The parenchymal blush (2) in the head of the pancreas reflects the high injection pressure required to force contrast past the stricture.

515. Cancer of the pancreas. An endoscopic retrograde cholangiogram reveals a grossly dilated common bile duct (1), intrahepatic biliary tree (2) and gall bladder (3). Note the blunt termination at the lower end of the bile duct caused by the pancreatic cancer. The prominent mucosal folds of the gall bladder are caused by oedema.

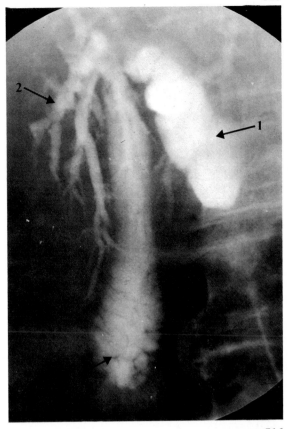

516. Cancer of the pancreas obstructing the lower end of the common bile duct caused this massive dilatation (arrowed).

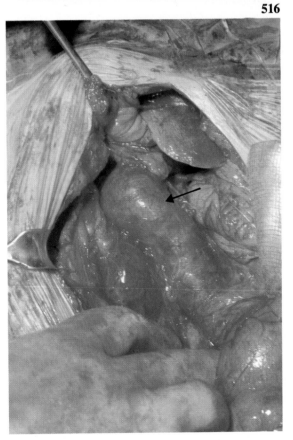

517. Cancer of the ampulla of Vater is an uncommon cause of common bile duct obstruction. Jaundice may be mild and intermittent. The tumour may bleed into the gastro-intestinal tract causing anaemia and a 'silver' stool. This barium meal examination shows a filling defect (arrowed) in the second part of the duodenum caused by cancer of the ampulla of Vater.

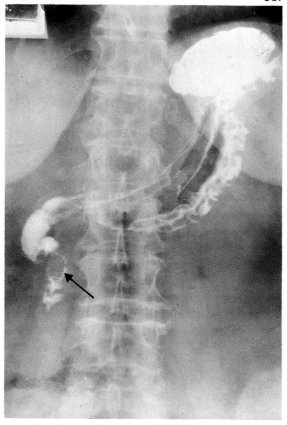

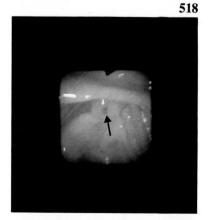

518. Ampulla of Vater (arrowed) is a nipple-like projection usually situated in the second part of the duodenum. The common bile duct and pancreatic duct drain via the ampulla of Vater into the duodenum. In this endoscopic picture bile is escaping from the ostium of the ampulla. A transverse fold of duodenal mucosa lies above it.

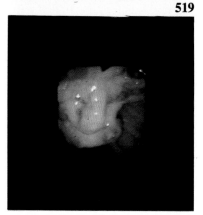

519. Cancer of the ampulla of Vater. The ampulla is usually enlarged with a necrotic surface which bleeds readily. This endoscopic picture shows a pale green slough covering an ampullary cancer. A cannula easily passed through this necrotic tissue to enter the common bile duct (**520**).

520. Cancer of the ampulla of Vater. An endoscopic retrograde cholangiogram from the patient illustrated in **519** shows a very dilated common bile duct (1) and intrahepatic biliary tree (2). Note the rounded obstruction (3) at the lower end of the common bile duct, due to the ampullary cancer.

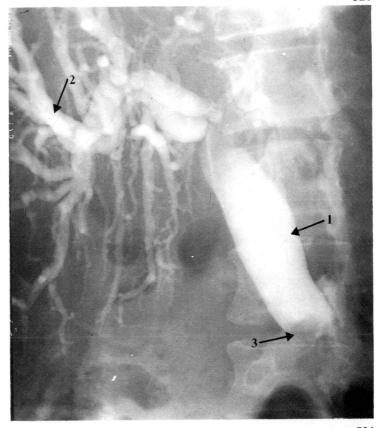

521. Pancreatic pseudocyst may obstruct the common bile duct. The appearance may be confused with a malignant bile duct stricture. However, extrinsic compression by a cyst causes stretching and displacement of the common bile duct (arrowed). The intrahepatic bile ducts are dilated.

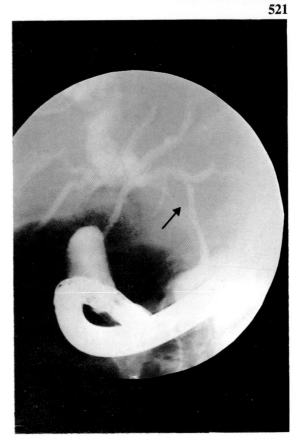

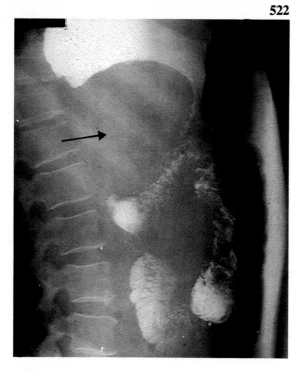

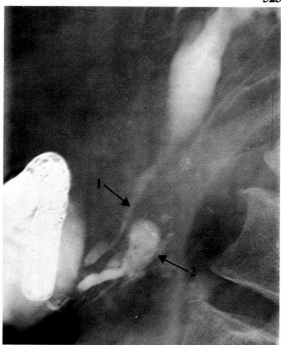

522. Pancreatic pseudocyst (arrowed) is revealed as a large retrogastric mass pushing the stomach forward in this barium meal examination.

523. Chronic pancreatitis may lead to a stricture of the lower end of the common bile duct and cholestasis. In contrast to a malignant obstruction, this stricture (1) is long and smoothly tapering. A short length of the pancreatic duct filled before the contrast entered a small pancreatic cyst (2). This x-ray of an endoscopic retrograde cholangio-pancreatogram was taken in the lateral projection.

524. Hodgkin's disease may rarely involve the main bile ducts and cause jaundice. This endoscopic retrograde cholangiogram shows obstruction of both the common bile duct (1) and pancreatic duct (2) by Hodgkin's deposits. Other causes of jaundice in Hodgkin's disease include haemolysis and an obscure intrahepatic cholestasis.

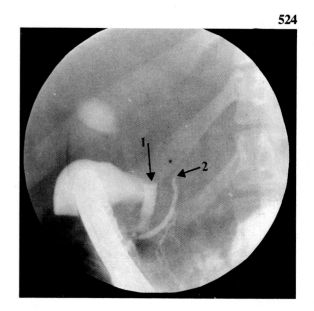

11. Gallstones

Gallstones are classified according to their predominant component as either *cholesterol* stones or *pigment* stones. Cholesterol gallstones are the commonest type encountered in the Western world. A small proportion are pigment gallstones. Pigment stones also develop in chronic haemolytic states, cirrhosis, recurrent biliary infections and in the Far East are associated with *Clonorchis sinensis* infestations.

525. Cholesterol gallstones are usually multiple, faceted and a greeny-yellow colour. They may contain varying amounts of calcium salts. Occasionally a single large gallstone is found in the gall bladder.

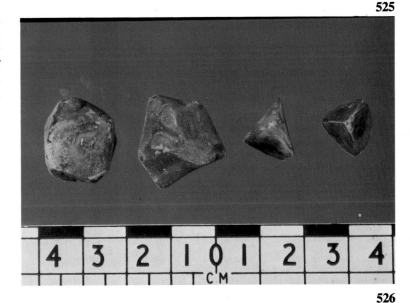

525

526. Pigment gallstones are generally small, round and a dark green or black colour. The gall bladder may contain hundreds of calculi. These pigment stones were removed from a patient with thalassaemia major (see **542**).

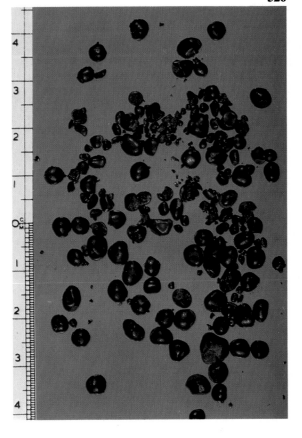

526

527. Calcified gallstones. A small proportion of gallstones contain sufficient calcium to make them radio-opaque in an abdominal x-ray. This plain x-ray (flat plate) shows the gall bladder full of stones with a peripheral ring of calcium.

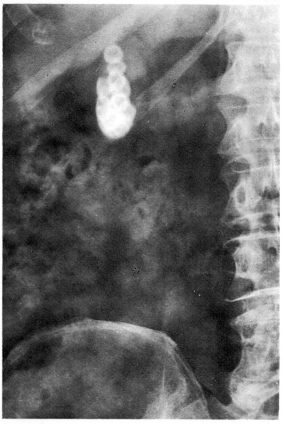

528. Calcified gallstones are occasionally laminated due to alternate deposition of layers of cholesterol and calcium salts.

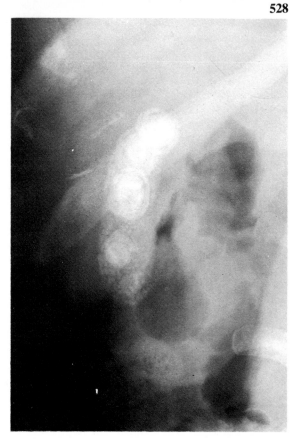

529. 'Mercedes Benz' sign. Rarely, the centre of a gallstone contains gas which shows as a stellate translucent pattern (arrowed) in an abdominal x-ray. In a search for the cause of this patient's abdominal pain a barium enema and intravenous pyelogram had been performed.

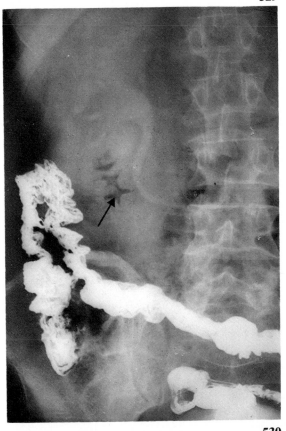

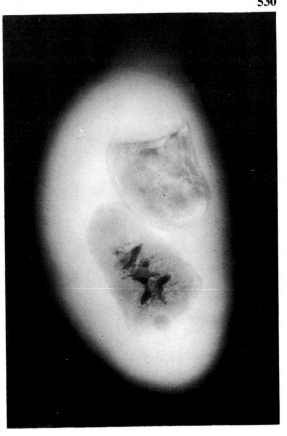

530. 'Mercedes Benz' sign. After cholecystectomy, an x-ray of the gall bladder specimen confirms that the translucent stellate pattern seen in **529** was due to gallstones.

531. Oral cholecystogram will demonstrate radio-lucent gallstones provided there is sufficient gall bladder function to concentrate the radio-opaque contrast medium. Tomography may be necessary. This cholecystogram shows at least five stones as lucent filling defects in the gall bladder.

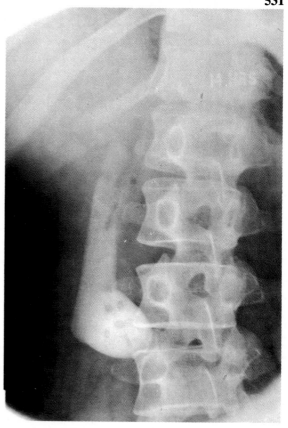

532. Oral cholecystogram. A fatty meal caused the gall bladder shown in **531** to contract. This is a sign of good gall bladder function. The calculi are seen more clearly.

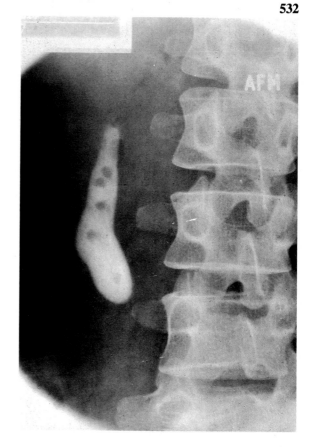

533. Intravenous cholangiogram may be used to opacify stones in the bile ducts and when the gall bladder fails to opacify in an oral cholecystogram. This x-ray shows two stones in the gall bladder (1). There are no calculi in the common bile duct (2). The contrast medium is draining freely into the duodenum (3).

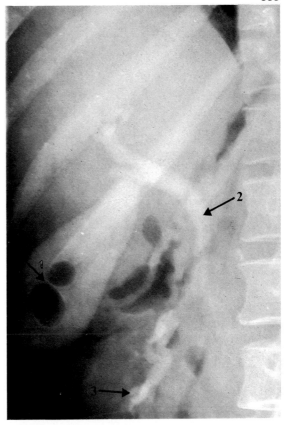

534. Floating gallstones (arrowed) are lying on the surface of a dense layer of contrast medium in the gall bladder. These calculi were only seen when the patient stood erect. Most stones are sufficiently dense to sink through the contrast medium.

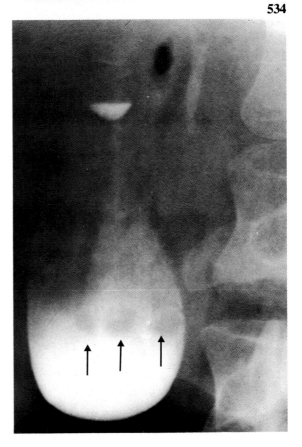

535. Gallstones. Occasionally an excessive amount of radio-opaque contrast can conceal stones in the biliary system. An early x-ray in this endoscopic retrograde cholangiogram shows a radiolucent stone in the gall bladder.

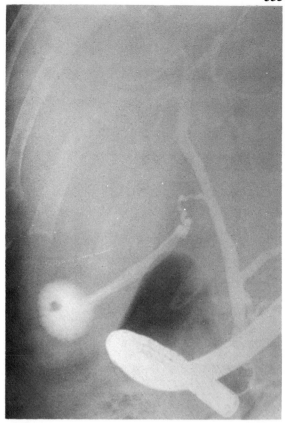

536. Gallstone shown in **535** is no longer visible in a later x-ray from the same examination. The stone is hidden by the dense contrast medium.

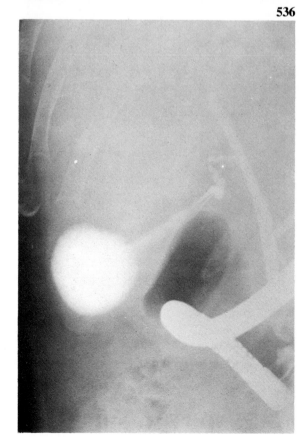

537. 'Phrygian cap' is a congenital malformation causing folding between the body and fundus (arrowed) of the gall bladder. Gall bladder function is normal. A 'phrygian cap' is of no significance but must not be confused with disease of the gall bladder in cholangiograms.

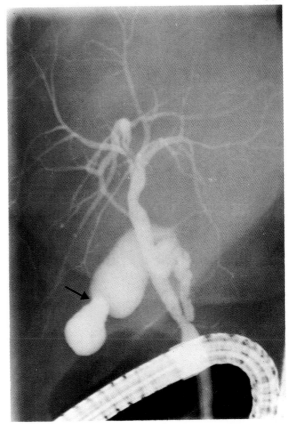

538

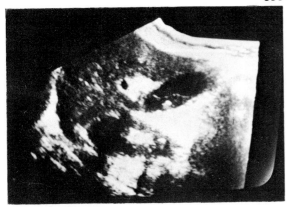

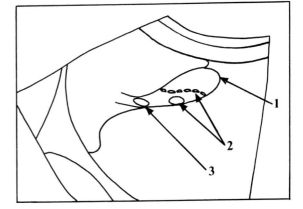

538. Acute cholecystitis usually follows impaction of a stone in the cystic duct. This grey-scale ultrasonogram shows a distended gall bladder (1) containing stones (2). A stone is impacted in the cystic duct (3). The inflamed and distended gall bladder causes abdominal pain and tenderness on palpation of the liver edge (Murphy's sign). Infection may develop causing a pyrexia. In severe cases the gall bladder is filled with pus (empyema of the gall bladder).

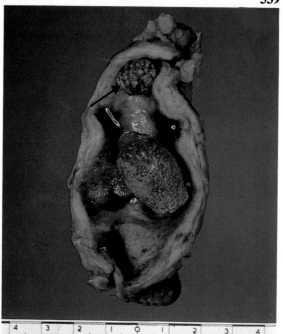

539. Chronic cholecystitis follows recurrent attacks of inflammation. The gall bladder wall is thickened and chronically inflamed. Several stones are present, one is obstructing the cystic duct (arrowed).

541

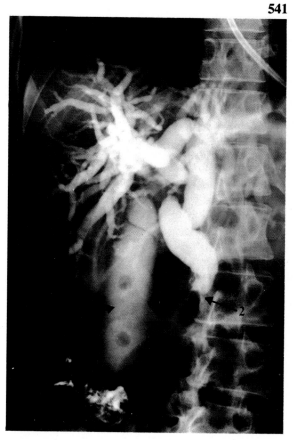

540

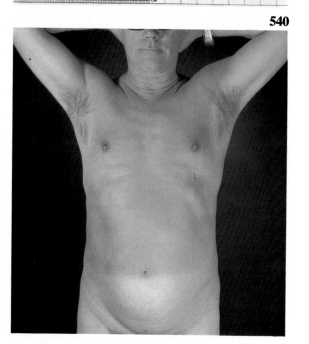

540. Gallstones in the common bile duct have usually migrated from the gall bladder. Biliary colic, cholangitis and cholestatic jaundice may develop. This patient became jaundiced after an attack of biliary colic while on holiday (he is suntanned). The serum bilirubin level was 11mg/100ml (187μmol/l).

541. Percutaneous cholangiogram from the patient in **540** shows stones in the gall bladder (1) and a stone (2) obstructing the lower end of a dilated bile duct.

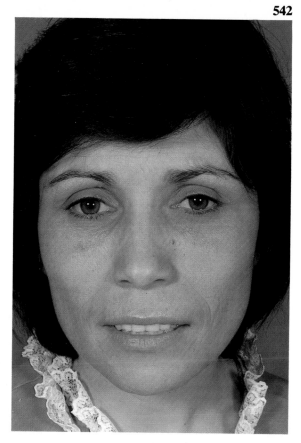

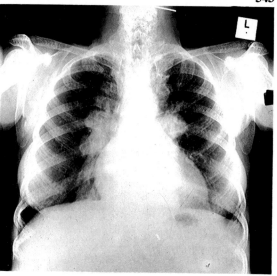

543. Thalassaemia. A chest x-ray from the patient in **542** shows circular shadows at the hila of both lungs. These are masses of erythropoietic tissue at the posterior ends of the ribs. The ribs show coarse trabeculation. The enlarged heart is due to iron overload in the myocardium.

542. Chronic haemolysis is associated with pigment gallstones, which may obstruct the common bile duct. This patient with thalassaemia major suddenly developed jaundice, itching, pale stools and dark urine. The serum bilirubin concentration was 19mg/100ml (323 ιmol/l). Note the prominent malar bones which are enlarged with erythropoietic tissue.

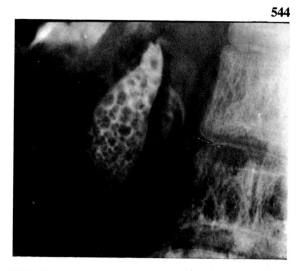

544. Thalassaemia. A percutaneous cholangiogram from the patient in **543** shows the gall bladder full of stones. The coarse trabeculation of the vertebral bones is due to the excessive erythropoiesis of a chronic haemolytic state. This is the clue that the calculi are probably pigment stones. The stones are shown in **526**.

545. Air in the biliary tree (1) is usually a consequence of biliary tract surgery, either a sphincterotomy or an anastomosis between the bile duct and the small intestine. Rarely, it is caused by infection with gas producing organisms such as *Clostridium welchii*. Air in the biliary tree may also follow the spontaneous passage of gallstones from the biliary tract into the gut. In this patient, the round shadow at the lower end of the air-filled common bile duct is a gallstone (2). The patient was suffering from biliary colic when the x-ray was taken. Note the fluid levels (3) in the surrounding 'sentinel' loops of bowel. Rarely, the passage of a large gallstone may cause intestinal obstruction ('gallstone ileus').

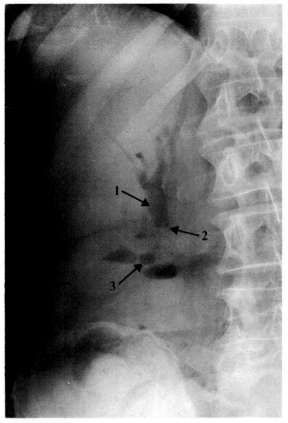

546. Cirrhotic patients have a high incidence of gallstones. The stones are predominantly of the pigment type. This endoscopic retrograde cholangiogram from a patient with cryptogenic cirrhosis shows radiolucent stones (arrowed) in the gall bladder.

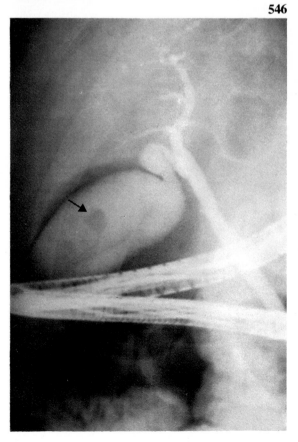

547. Pancreatitis may be caused by a gallstone (1) at the ampulla of Vater obstructing the pancreatic duct (2). This endoscopic retrograde cholangiogram was performed soon after an attack of acute pancreatitis.

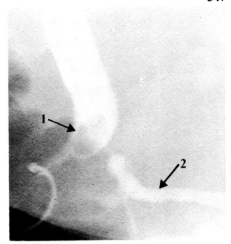

548. Cystic duct remnant (1) after cholecystectomy may be very long if the cystic duct is inserted low down the common bile duct (2). Symptoms are uncommon. However stones may develop in a long cystic duct stump and result in recurrent attacks of cholangitis.

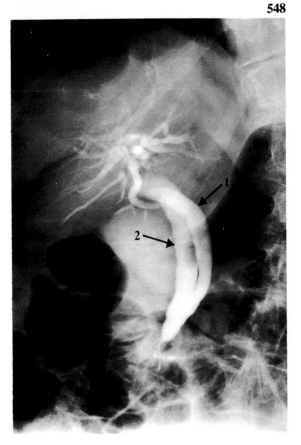

549. Retained bile duct stones after biliary surgery may cause persistent jaundice, cholangitis and biliary fistulae. This patient remained jaundiced after cholecystectomy and leaked about 500ml of bile each day through a wound drain. The endoscopic retrograde cholangiogram shows a dilated biliary tree obstructed by a single stone (1). Note the cystic duct remnant (2) and the wound drain (3) through which bile was leaking.

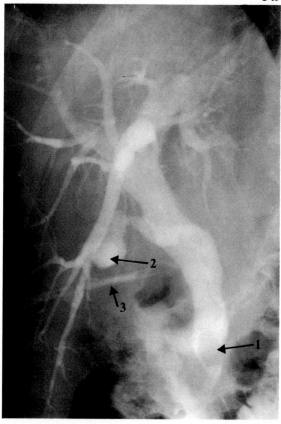

550. Retained bile duct stone shown in **549** was removed by endoscopic sphincterotomy. Cholesterol was the principal component of this oval calculus.

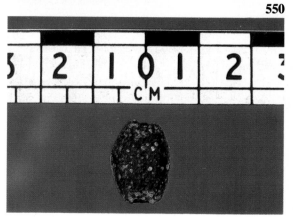

551. Retained bile duct stones. This patient became jaundiced after a cholecystectomy. A percutaneous cholangiogram shows three stones (1) obstructing the lower end of a dilated common bile duct. A long cystic duct remnant (2) was present.

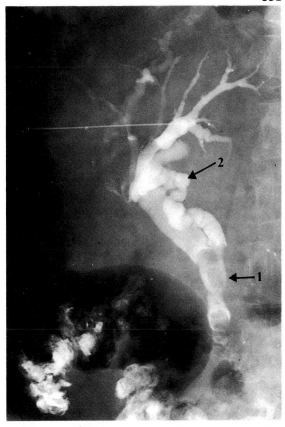

552. Intrahepatic gallstones usually follow prolonged biliary obstruction, due to a bile duct stricture or sclerosing cholangitis. In the Far East they are associated with *Clonorchis sinensis* infestation. Small, gritty, dark-green or black pigment gallstones are the usual finding. This operative cholangiogram from a patient with a benign post-cholecystectomy biliary stricture shows multiple intrahepatic gallstones (arrowed).

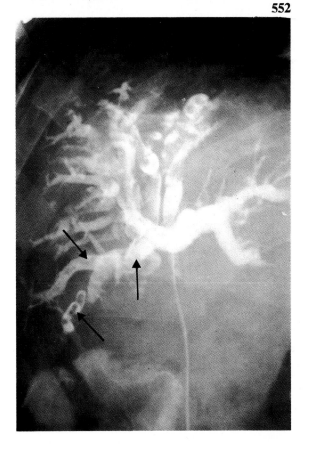

553. Solitary duodenal diverticulum at the ampulla of Vater is associated with gallstones. In this patient the ampulla of Vater was hidden inside the diverticulum. The endoscopic picture shows bile escaping from the mouth of the diverticulum.

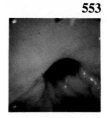

554. Solitary duodenal diverticulum in **553** has been filled with contrast medium (arrowed). It is situated in the second part of the duodenum which is filled with air.

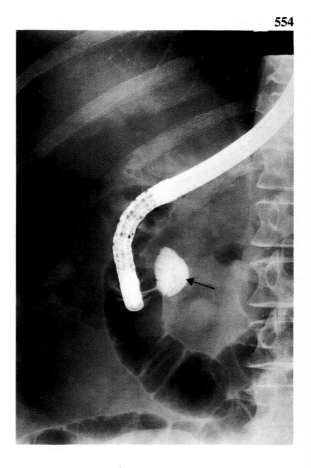

Index